massage

in essence

massage

in essence

Nicola Jenkins

Hodder Arnold

A MEMBER OF THE HODDER HEADLINE GROUP

Orders: please contact Bookpoint Ltd, 130 Milton Park, Abingdon, Oxon OX14 4SB. Telephone: (44) 01235 827720. Fax: (44) 01235 400454. Lines are open from 9.00 – 5.00, Monday to Saturday, with a 24 hour message answering service. You can also order through our website www.hoddereducation.co.uk

If you have any comments to make about this, or any of our other titles, please send them to
educationenquiries@hodder.co.uk

British Library Cataloguing in Publication Data
A catalogue record for this title is available from the British Library

ISBN-10: 0 340 91678 8
ISBN-13: 978 0 340 91678 0

First Edition Published 2006
Impression number   10 9 8 7 6 5 4 3 2 1
Year   2011 2010 2009 2008 2007 2006

Copyright © 2006 Nicola Jenkins

Hodder Headline's policy is to use papers that are natural, renewable and recyclable products and made from wood grown in sustainable forests. The logging and manufacturing processes are expected to conform to the environmental regulations of the country of origin.

Cover photo from Frank P. Wartenberg/Photonica/Getty Images
Artwork by Oxford Designers and Illustrators Ltd
Typeset by Servis Filmsetting Ltd, Manchester

Printed in Great Britain for Hodder Arnold, an imprint of Hodder Education, a member of the Hodder Headline Group, 338 Euston Road, London NW1 3BH by CPI Bath

acknowledgements

Thank you to all the usual suspects for their support and encouragement in the development of this manuscript, especially to Tamsin Smith, who approached me with the initial idea and was so encouraging as we developed the concepts for the series; to Andrew James for his ongoing enthusiasm and his help in refining my ideas; and to Claire Baranowski for additional questions for the collection. Particular thanks are also owed this time to my mum, Carol Jenkins, my mother-in-law, Greta Stewart, and to my husband, Alan Stewart, for childcare above and beyond the call of duty – Hannah thanks you all very much for entertaining her while I wrote. I have also written this with Rachel Haffner in mind: we have known each other over 20 years, we both left our dignity at the hospital door when we had children and she still cannot stand the thought of letting me massage her in case I see any cellulite (she has none). Last, but not least, I would like to thank long-term friend, fellow massage tutor and life coach, Patricia Bryce, for motivational postcards, phone calls and text messages that kept arriving just when I needed a swift kick.

The authors and publishers would like to thank the following for the permission to use the following photographs in this volume:

Picture credits: **pp. 4** Musée d'Histoire de la Medecine, Paris, France, Archives Charmet/Bridgeman Art Library, **pp. 5** Dave Bartruff, Inc./Corbis, **pp. 16** Anthea Sieveking/Wellcome Photo Library; **pp. 24** (both) Dr P. Marazzi/Science Photo Library, **pp. 48** Courtesy DK Profashion, **pp. 49** Courtesy Natural Living

All other photographs © Carl Drury

With thanks to Minna and Stuart, our models, and to Images Model Agency.

contents

understanding massage

When your friends and family find out that you are starting a massage class, they may ask, 'What is there to understand about massage? It's not like a back rub can really do anything but ease stiff muscles, is it?' The truth, as you are about to find out, is very different. Massage can help you in so many ways, and, as you embark on this adventure, you will find out that easing painfully tight muscles is just the beginning.

introduction

For many, massage is the first step they take in a long journey of self-discovery, full of interesting landmarks:

꙰ The first time you have a treatment – and perhaps hesitate when you think about the price you are paying and the length of time it takes. Afterwards, you wonder why you did not try massage earlier, or how often you can afford to have treatments, because you deserve to feel that good always.

꙰ The first time you take your clothes off for a treatment (from a friend or from a professional therapist) and the associated worries about your body's appearance (or whether you have nice underwear on). As you get more comfortable, you stop worrying about how your body looks undressed and start worrying about how quickly you can remove your clothes and get on the massage table to get maximum treatment time.

꙰ The first time you notice that you feel different after giving or receiving a treatment. Maybe you are more relaxed, you can sleep better or suddenly the aches and pains have disappeared. Perhaps there might be something in this…

꙰ The first course you take in massage because you have decided that you want to learn more and that somehow it might signal a change in your health, how you feel about yourself, your life or your work.

There's a lot of history to the use of massage. Hippocrates recommended its application on a daily basis as being beneficial to health. There are hieroglyphic images on the walls of the tombs of Egypt, showing body and foot massage taking place. The term 'massage' has its roots in both the Greek and Arabic languages, from which it can be translated as 'kneading' and 'gently pressing', respectively. In parts of the world, whole therapeutic disciplines have developed which emphasize the benefits of touch and massage – shiatsu in Japan, huna in Hawaii, Ayurvedic treatments in India (including Indian head massage), Tui na, acupressure and Thai massages, all with their distinctive styles and methods of application. You may be more familiar with reflexology, aromatherapy and stone therapy – all of which developed as specialist forms of massage.

massage in essence

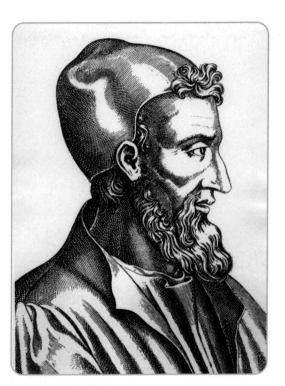

The Ancient Greek medicinal practitioner Galen recommended massage for health and well-being

As well as differences in the application of massage around the world, it is also interesting to note that people learn these treatments in different ways. For example, in Japan, many children grow up learning how to give basic shiatsu treatments to their parents and siblings. While massage is increasing in popularity in the UK, we have not yet reached a point where it is a regular occurrence in every household. It is more common now, however, and massage methods are taught to expectant parents as part of their preparation for labour and birth. Although baby massage is actively encouraged as part of the parent–child bonding process, there is still room for improvement and for treatment to continue beyond the cradle. There are still distinct groups who do not regularly receive the therapeutic benefits of touch outside of a

sexual relationship. This may account, in part, for why massage is still viewed by many in Britain as being overtly sexual and more than slightly risqué.

However, with the increasing number of courses in massage, not only in further education colleges, but also as part of university degree programmes, there has been a subsequent increase in the amount of research being carried out into the effects of massage on the physical, mental and emotional states of humans and animals. Chapter 2 concentrates on the physical benefits of massage, but recent research at the Touch Institute at the University of Miami, Florida (www.miami.edu/touch-research/home.html – accessed 27 November 2005), into some of the more unusual effects of massage in controlled studies, has unearthed the following:

- Parents massaging asthmatic children were able to improve their children's peak airflow (the maximum amount of air flowing into and out of the lungs) and lung functioning, reduce anxiety and noticeably reduce the levels of stress hormones (cortisol, which keeps blood sugar levels high in order to give you the energy you need to cope with stressful situations). They also reported feeling less anxious themselves.

- Children with attention deficit hyperactivity disorder who were given twice-weekly massages for a month were reported by their teachers as being able to concentrate for longer on assigned tasks and as being less hyperactive in class.

- Bulimic adolescent girls who received massage twice a week for five weeks reported an improved body image, feeling less anxious and depressed, and were also discovered to have reduced

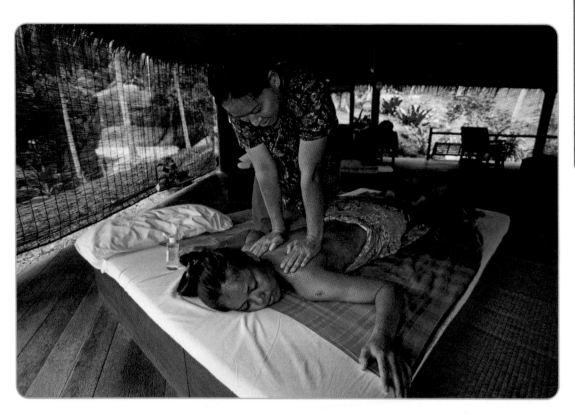

Thai massage has developed its own distinctive style

cortisol levels and improved dopamine and serotonin levels (these are neurotransmitters, substances used by the nervous system to transmit messages effectively: dopamine is involved in helping you sleep better and serotonin is involved in helping you feel happier – serotonin is usually the substance that needs to be replaced or enhanced if someone is depressed).

❧ One month of regular massage for children with diabetes helped to bring blood sugar levels down to a normal level, improved the children's ability to stick to required dietary regimes (and their willingness to do so) and improved anxiety levels in both the children and their parents.

❧ Adults who received massage were found to have significant changes to the electrical activity within their brains, all indicating improved alertness. They were then set mathematics problems, which they were able to complete faster and more accurately as a result of the treatments. Anxiety and stress levels were noticeably lower at the end of the five-week testing period.

❧ Massage during labour, for just 15 minutes in each hour of labour, resulted in a shorter hospital stay, shorter labour and less depressed mood in the mother.

❧ Cravings, nervous habits and the number of cigarettes smoked were decreased by using self-massage whenever a craving was experienced in the individual attempting to reduce their smoking habit.

One of the most interesting pieces of recent research carried out by the Touch Institute reports on the benefits of massage to the person providing the massage. A group of elderly volunteers, half of whom were taught infant massage, were assessed after a month of either giving treatment or receiving a massage themselves. At the end of the month, those who had given massage were able to report being less anxious and depressed and felt noticeably happier. They were also noted as having lower pulse rates, lower cortisol levels and improved self-esteem, and had made significant positive changes to their social activities.

With massage developing over the centuries in so many different parts of the world, there are distinct differences in the way a treatment is carried out. The following are very brief descriptions of the more common forms of massage available in the UK. More detailed descriptions will be available from your local practitioners.

Massage styles made simple

Massage style	Description
Acupressure	Based on traditional Chinese medicine, this form of massage uses strong pressure applied to specific points (identical to those used in acupuncture) in order to improve health, posture, flexibility and much more.
Aromatherapy	Combines massage (usually the techniques of holistic or Swedish massage, although other forms of massage are also incorporated) with the use of essential oils (concentrated extracts from plants). Self-help and home use of the essential oils between treatments usually involves adding essential oils to bath or shower products, as inhalations or to vaporize in a room.
Ayurvedic massage	Based on the concept that prana, or life energy, flows through 107 marma points situated around the body, and that massage can affect the flow of this prana. The client's dosha (the way in which the life energy is expressed) is identified according to Ayurvedic principles, following which suitable oils (including, occasionally, essential oils) are chosen to enhance the treatment.
Chavutti Thirumal	A variety of Ayurvedic massage in which the practitioner uses a rope to help them balance as they use their feet to apply the massage strokes to their clients as the clients lie on the floor.
Deep-tissue massage	Often linked with acupressure, this involves a very deep massage, with specific pressure techniques, in order to aid the recovery of musculoskeletal problems, as well as supporting the health of other internal organs; it tends to improve muscle tone, increase circulation and improve flexibility and posture.
Holistic massage	The term 'holistic' is usually defined as taking into consideration the body, mind, emotions, spirit and environment of the person receiving the treatment. As a result, a holistic massage is usually seen as one in which the therapist adapts the movements they know (or the routine they are familiar with) in order to treat the

Massage style	Description
	specific needs of the client they are treating on that day. Holistic massage tends to be based around the movements learned in Swedish or therapeutic massage.
Huna	Originating in Hawaii, this form of massage involves a two-hour treatment, designed to encourage a more positive outlook in the client, especially with regard to themselves and their actions.
Indian head massage/ Champissage™	Originally applied only to the hair and scalp in order to maintain the health of the hair and skin in this area, its techniques have been developed, resulting in a very relaxing treatment to the head, neck, shoulders and upper back.
Manual lymphatic drainage	A specialist form of massage which involves particularly light and gentle strokes in order to encourage lymphatic vessels close to the skin to release toxins and promote the removal of toxins and oedema from the body. This is particularly useful as a supporting treatment following operations such as mastectomies, where the lymph nodes may be affected and oedema is likely to develop.
Reflexology	A very detailed pressure massage of the feet and/or hands, designed to stimulate reflex points, which, in turn, will affect the health of the body and encourage a return to balance and optimum health, as well as promoting a feeling of profound well-being.
Remedial massage	A specialist treatment designed to focus on muscles which are overstrained, overstretched and in pain as a result of overuse. The practitioner concentrates on the damaged or painful muscles.
Shiatsu	Originating in Japan, this form of massage concentrates on improving the flow of chi through the body by using the hands, fingers and palms to press on the acupressure points relating to joints and muscles. As with acupressure, some of the movements are very specific and require the practitioner to have a deep and thorough understanding of the meridians (the pathways in the body along which vital energy is said to flow).
Sports massage	Used before sporting events or exercise as a means of warming up the muscles effectively, and after events to warm down, as well as to identify any injury or damage and to take simple steps to relax the muscles, to prevent injury or muscle strain and to speed up the rate of recovery.
Stone therapy	Massage using hot and cold stones (lava and marble stones, respectively) as part of the treatment. Some therapists incorporate the use of essential oils in the treatment, although the massage treatment is already enhanced by the use of temperature and the change in pressure available from using the stones.
Swedish (or therapeutic) massage	Uses specific techniques – including effleurage, petrissage, kneading, tapotement – to treat the soft tissues of the body (muscles, tendons, ligaments and skin). Movements are primarily towards the heart, in order to improve the circulation of blood and lymph, as well as to reduce muscle tension and encourage flexibility.

Massage style	Description
Thai massage	As well as being a very firm style of massage, this involves extensive stretches to enhance and improve joint and muscle flexibility for the client. Therapists will frequently use feet, elbows and knees when they work.
Tui na	Acupressure-style massage which originated in China and uses the same diagnostic tools as acupuncture; however, treatment involves pressure applied with thumbs, fingers, hands or elbows to specific points, as well as occasional stretches and manipulation of joints.

FAQs: About massage in general

I am not sure I like the idea of taking off my clothes to be massaged. Do I have to remove them for the treatment?

Yes and no. On-site massage is a seated version of massage which is usually carried out over your clothes and which is most often provided in an office environment. Shiatsu is also carried out over your clothes, and in reflexology you only need to remove your shoes and socks. However, this book concentrates on therapeutic or holistic massage. For these types of massage, it is expected that you will remove some clothing for the treatment, although the therapist will take very close care to ensure that you feel safe and warm while the treatment is in progress. If you are learning massage, you will be expected to remove your clothing at appropriate points during the course; however, your tutor will be emphasizing the importance of towel management (see page 40) and how you can use large towels to maintain your own privacy and that of your classmates when undressing.

What would be your advice about treating people of the opposite sex?

This is something that professional massage therapists have to consider very carefully when they start to plan how they are going to work, as there is room for misunderstanding where massage is concerned – sometimes it is seen as an overture to sexual relations. The short answer to this question is that if you are worried or concerned about treating either a particular person or a group of people in general, then you should refrain from doing something that makes you uncomfortable.

I think that it is a valuable learning opportunity to treat as many different people as you can; each body is unique and will exhibit different patterns of stress, muscle tension, congestion and injury. The more variety you experience, the easier it will become for you to tell the difference between what is healthy and what is not when you massage a new person. What remains, then, is to work as safely as possible, taking into consideration any

Throughout this book, and especially in the massage routines themselves, I will be mentioning specific muscles by name. These are always accompanied by line drawings so that you can recognize where they appear. The names (and the Latin in general) are introduced so that you can start to become more familiar with what some people find to be the hardest aspect of learning about anatomy and physiology –

picking up a new language at the same time. Remember that really all you are learning is geography, in a way that allows you to be specific when describing where you are working and why (if you know what the muscles do or what their names mean). Learning anatomy and physiology is something you will need to do if you want to proceed further than an introductory course in massage.

contraindication to treatment (see chapter 3) and your own personal safety.

Remember, although the assumption tends to be that it is female therapists who are at risk from male clients, the opposite can also be true.

What type of person makes the best massage therapist?
Someone who loves to massage. You do not have to be outgoing and you do not need to have lots of experience or a brilliant CV; you just need to be patient, to enjoy the act of massaging, to be willing to learn what someone's body is trying to tell you and to spend time practising what you know. If you go on to qualify as a massage therapist, you will need to spend a lot of time practising as well as studying anatomy and physiology.

You also need to have short nails, clean hands, be physically fit enough to carry out

the treatment you are trained to do and know when to refer someone on, either to another practitioner or to their doctor (because the situation they are presenting with exceeds your knowledge and experience).

Does massage require a lot of physical strength?
No. Although most people like a firm treatment when they have a massage, if you know how to use your body weight effectively, you will not have to build up your upper body strength at all. If someone you are treating asks you to press harder (and this is difficult for you), you can usually get a better result by lowering your massage table slightly, locking your elbows for most of the movements, keeping your back straight when working and lunging into the movements from your hips.

the benefits
of massage

chapter

Have you ever stopped to consider what the world might be like if we could find some way to get every person on the planet a massage at least once a week? To begin with, we would all be distinctly healthier, sleep and work more effectively and most likely greet any problems life throws at us with a calmer disposition.

The benefits of massage have been referred to in traditional medicine for centuries.

Hippocrates recommended daily massage with herbal infusions for healthy living; foot massage appears in illustrations on the walls of many an Egyptian tomb; Ayurvedic treatments in India are often applied through the medium of massage; the list goes on. But what does massage actually do to us? What are the real, tangible benefits to the practice of massage?

Benefits to the skin

As soon as you start a massage, you are already beginning to benefit the body by taking care of the health of the skin and improving its appearance. Using a vegetable oil, such as sweet almond or grapeseed oil, will provide the skin with a new source of valuable nutrients, vitamins and minerals. Regular massage with the right kinds of vegetable oils can encourage the skin to regenerate effectively, will remove dry, scaly skin from the surface (so that the skin appears younger and fresher) and will help to improve the production of sebum – the skin's natural form of lubrication.

Regular massage also helps to improve the skin's ability to excrete waste products via sweat, with the result that more sweat is produced. This is one of the reasons that a massage therapist will often tell you to increase the amount of water you drink following a treatment: if you drink more water you will not be dehydrated as a result of the water you have lost via sweat, and you will be able to effectively excrete any remaining toxins that have been mobilized as a result of the treatment. (These are removed from the body via your kidneys as urine; often you will need to urinate shortly after a massage and

11

you may find that your urine is more concentrated than usual.)

Using a lotion or a mineral oil (such as baby oil) is also helpful, adding another barrier to protect the skin from the elements. Both these products tend to sit on the surface of the skin, so while they are useful on occasion for massage, vegetable oils are a preferred option.

Massage, especially if it is fairly vigorous, helps to improve circulation to the skin and underlying muscles. You will see this quite quickly in the way the skin becomes warmer and pinker to the touch as you continue to massage. Improving the circulation to the skin also helps to bring the skin and underlying tissues more nutrients (carried around the body via the blood). Massage also encourages blood and lymph (plasma which

has escaped from the blood system into surrounding tissues) to return to the cardiovascular system, reducing some types of oedema, or swelling, in the process.

Careful, regular massage can also help to loosen and stretch scar tissue, especially if it is deep scarring. Massaging in and around areas of recent scarring, however, is best left in the hands of a professional therapist, as you need to ensure that the scars are properly healed and will not break open when massaged. Once the tissue is sufficiently healed to be massaged, gentle massage can be beneficial: by loosening and stretching the tissues in the area, you can improve circulation to the scar tissue, so healing occurs faster; you can also help to mobilize the tissue so that the person's skin and underlying muscle returns to full flexibility.

Benefits to the muscles

The benefits of massage to the muscles are probably the most obvious; the key ones being pain relief and the reduction of muscle tension.

When a muscle goes into spasm it contracts painfully, limiting movement (as it will not stretch out or return to its resting size or shape easily). When it contracts, it often clamps down on nearby nerves or nerve endings (hence we feel pain), and often on nearby blood vessels as well – so circulation is limited to the muscle and to nearby tissues (such as skin). As a result, we often develop a condition that can spiral out of control – we feel pain, movement is limited, the area is cold and feels hard to the touch. Massage gently helps to warm the area and the underlying muscles; the improved circulation provides additional warmth and nutrients, as well as removing the waste products which have been

generated (possibly as a result of the muscle working too hard and then going into spasm). As the muscles relax, the pain stops.

Regular massage can also help to maintain and improve muscle tone. This can be invaluable if you have a massage either before or after exercise. Massage before exercise will warm up your muscles properly and can reduce the chance of injury. Massage after exercise functions as a warm-down, and can also help to assess and remedy any injury you might have sustained.

An additional benefit to improving muscle tone is that posture is often improved as a result. Improved posture not only helps you to feel more positive, but also improves the effectiveness of your muscles and reduces the risk of pain or discomfort returning as quickly as before.

Benefits to the cardiovascular system

Each time the heart contracts it pushes blood along the arteries towards the skin, muscles, tissues and other organs of the body. As blood reaches these destinations, it enters into smaller and smaller blood vessels until it reaches the capillaries – tiny vessels whose walls are only one cell thick. When blood leaves the capillaries, it enters the veins to return to the heart (where it will begin this journey again); however, there is no pump such as the heart to push the blood along the veins. Venous flow (the passage of blood along the veins back to the heart) is almost exclusively managed as a result of muscle contractions taking place near the veins. As the muscles contract, so they press blood towards the heart. When this normal activity is slowed down, possibly by injury, illness or inactivity (and this would include standing still for long periods of time), the rate of blood circulation slows down and you can get blood pooling in certain areas, with swelling resulting. In severe cases, varicose veins can develop. One of the most valuable benefits of massage is that it aids venous flow: the pressure applied in massage imitates muscle contraction and helps to improve circulation.

As an area is warmed during massage the underlying blood vessels are encouraged to dilate so that more blood can come into the tissues, bringing fresh nutrients and more oxygen, and getting rid of waste products.

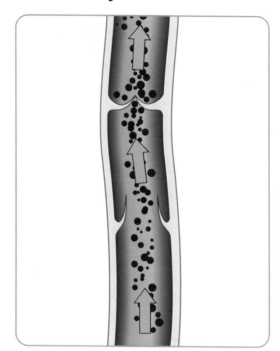

Structure of a vein

The pressure and speed of the massage can also help to soothe or stimulate circulation; someone who needs warming up would benefit from a vigorous treatment (which would also help to stimulate the mind and motivate them to get things done). Someone with high blood pressure, high stress levels or who is very anxious would benefit from a slow, soothing treatment to calm their nerves and slow down the heart rate.

Benefits to the skeleton

Improving the circulation of blood also helps to improve the general health of the bones in the body. In this way, massage acts in a similar fashion to exercise – both activities encourage calcium in the blood to be absorbed by the bones, thereby strengthening them and helping to reduce the risk of degenerative diseases, such as osteoarthritis or osteoporosis (where the bones become very brittle and break easily).

Regular massage which concentrates on the muscles, tendons (these attach muscles to bone) and ligaments (these link bones to other bones and maintain the stability of a joint) around joints in the skeleton also helps to enhance the health of these attachments, reduce any pain in the area and improve mobility.

Benefits to the endocrine system

The endocrine system is the name we give to a group of organs that make hormones – chemical messengers that move around the body via the blood to target organs (organs which respond to the chemical message), where they elicit a response. Hormones are released when there is a change in your body's internal or external environment and the body needs to respond to that change in order to stay healthy. Hormones are involved in maintaining stable conditions within the body and are responsible for many of the small, precise changes the body needs to function healthily. For instance, hormones govern changes in blood pressure, blood sugar levels, blood calcium levels, body temperature, growth, your response to danger and much more. By improving the blood flow, massage also helps hormones to reach their target organs more quickly.

Massage also helps to:

- lower blood sugar levels by increasing the ability of cells to absorb sugar;
- relax the subject, so the output of stress hormones, such as adrenaline, noradrenaline and cortisol are all lowered;
- reduce the effects that stress will have on the functioning of other hormones, in particular those related to the reproductive system (oestrogen, progesterone and testosterone are all affected);
- stabilize the metabolic rate (the rate at which the body produces and uses energy); this is also governed by hormones, in this case by the hormones produced in the thyroid gland, notably thyroxine.

Benefits to the digestive system

Massage helps to support the digestive system by mimicking peristalsis, the wave-like muscle contractions which move material through the intestines. Regular massage can help to regulate bowel movements in a number of ways. Deep, precise massage movements, such as petrissage, can aid the removal of faecal material that has remained in the large intestine for a long time (see pages 115–16 for a sample routine). Gentle treatments are also

the benefits of massage

excellent at soothing the bowels where the symptoms of irritable bowel syndrome (IBS), including diarrhoea, are experienced. Abdominal massage of this kind is extremely effective, very relaxing and can be enjoyed at all ages; using massage to relieve colic and constipation is a key benefit of baby massage. Because it is so comforting, abdominal massage is particularly good to support people with stress-related conditions such as ulcers, and eating disorders such as bulimia or anorexia. In all these cases, the people in question may be reluctant at first to receive massage in this area, especially if they do not feel comfortable exposing their body; however, you can encourage them to try massaging themselves in this way as it will help to stimulate a feeling of well-being.

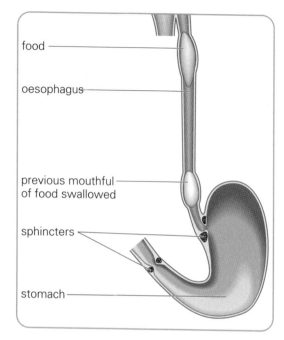

food

oesophagus

previous mouthful of food swallowed

sphincters

stomach

Peristalsis in the digestive system

Benefits to the reproductive system

Massage benefits the reproductive system at all stages of one's reproductive life. Regular massage – especially of the lower back and abdomen – can help to regulate menstrual periods throughout a woman's life and reduce menopausal symptoms as she reaches the end of her reproductive cycle. At this time in her life, regular massage is particularly effective at reducing any anxiety or unhappiness a woman may feel, improving sleep, reducing the effects of hot flushes, limiting night sweats, easing aching joints and improving the quality of the skin and nails, which can sometimes get very dry at this time.

Massage is particularly useful at relieving the pain associated with menstrual periods, endometriosis and labour. It is now an accepted and expected part of any antenatal class and is an invaluable skill for birthing partners in the delivery room.

Massage's sometimes less than respectable reputation also hints at its effectiveness at aiding fertility and sexual receptivity. While massage has been, and occasionally still is, used as a cover for prostitution, the reason for this cannot be denied – massage is extremely good at relaxing the individual, helping them to become more aware of their body's health and well-being. This, in turn, is likely to make the person more receptive to their loved one if sexual disinterest is an issue. With respect to fertility, studies carried out by Alice Domar, Director of Women's Health Services at Harvard's Mind-Body Medical Institute, highlight the links between stress, depression and sub-fertility. Her research shows depression to be more closely linked with infertility than anxiety; and also demonstrates that when couples with long-term fertility issues (having been unable to conceive for years, despite medical support and intervention) attended a mind-body infertility programme (consisting of visualization exercises, relaxation techniques, such as massage, and detailed support with respect to diet and lifestyle issues), there was an impressive figure of 44 per cent of delegates managing to conceive within six months of following the programme.

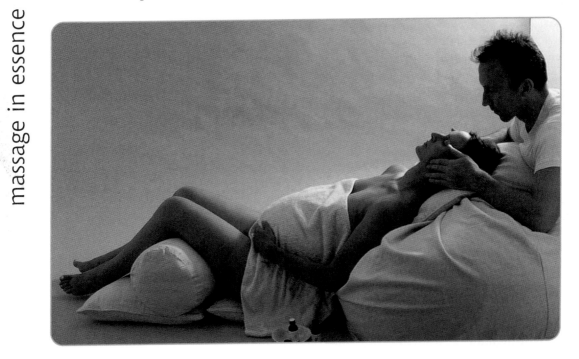

Massage can help reduce some of the side effects of pregnancy

Benefits to the mind and nervous system

The effectiveness of massage in the relief of stress and stress-related conditions is a good indication of just how much it has to offer the mind and the nervous system generally. Massage provides a profound sense of well-being, and, depending on the speed, pressure and frequency of treatment can be either stimulating or sedating. Clients receiving regular massage will emphasize its pain-relieving effects, its ability to improve sleep and motivation, and to relieve other, less tangible, symptoms of stress.

On a purely physical level, massage works on the neuromuscular junctions – the points at which a nerve enters a muscle. Regular massage enhances the effects of the neurotransmitters (the chemical messages a nerve sends to a muscle which instruct it to contract), meaning that the muscles can contract more quickly and effectively. The result? Your responses become faster.

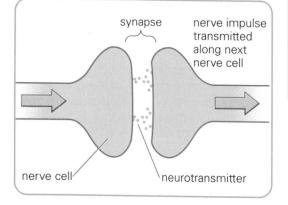

A nerve synapse

Work carried out on a muscle or group of muscles that are in spasm will relieve trapped nerves, which in turn will provide pain relief. It will also improve the blood circulation so that the nerves will receive all the nutrients they need to work effectively.

the benefits of massage

casestudy: Raynaud's syndrome

Jessica worked as a deputy head teacher at a large secondary school – a job she loved but found very demanding, both personally and professionally. Although there was a family history of Raynaud's syndrome, she did not develop it herself until the term her school was facing its Ofsted inspection. Raynaud's is an unusual disorder in which the small blood vessels in the person's extremities – usually the hands and feet – constrict for no apparent reason. The flesh in the area turns very pale and cold and does not respond normally to warmth or cold, so the hands and feet can feel as if they are freezing even on a very warm day. In Jessica's case, the problem was most noticeable in her hands and forearms, although the skin colouring and temperature returned to normal above the elbow.

The treatment on Jessica involved effleurage and kneading, primarily. Because her condition was stress-related, it also meant that she needed to relax completely (or as far as possible) before the work began on her hands and arms. This meant that each time she had a treatment (once a week for six weeks, at which time the sessions became less frequent), she received a full body treatment, in which we started by working on her back. This meant that by the time she turned over to have the fronts of her legs and arms and her face massaged, she was feeling very sleepy and comfortable. Jessica found the facial massage the most relaxing part of the treatment, so I taught her how to do a simple facial massage herself, which she could manage daily when she was applying her moisturizer in the morning and at night. Within two weeks she was pleased to report that not only was she far calmer during the day as a result, but she was also sleeping better and felt that she looked younger too. The Raynaud's was very slow to respond to massage, although it did make some difference. Jessica found that having the treatments made her far more aware of her body and she began to realize when she was going to have problems with her hands and forearms. She learnt that if she caught it at the right time, ran her hands under warm water and then massaged them herself with simple effleurage movements, she could reduce the associated pain and reduce the length of time during which her circulation gave her trouble.

FAQs: About the benefits of massage

My granny has very poor circulation and you mention that vigorous massage will improve circulation. I am a little worried about being vigorous as she is rather frail.
Any form of massage, even gentle effleurage alone, will improve circulation. In these circumstances, it is far more effective to be gentle, to carry out the treatment regularly and to use heat as part of the treatment. Try warming the oil that you use to massage her with, cover her with warm towels while she is having the treatment and make sure she keeps warm for a good couple of hours afterwards – often your body temperature will drop during a treatment.

Can massage help me lose weight?
Only as part of a calorie-controlled diet. What massage can do is help to tone up your muscles, reduce oedema (so any unwanted swelling is minimized), reduce your appetite and make your bowel habits more regular. Having said that, if you are the person doing the massages and you are doing a lot of treatments, especially ones which are very energetic (maybe a lot of cellulite treatments), then you will be using up so much energy that you stand a good chance of losing some weight in the process.

Do cellulite treatments really work?
Yes (see page 92 for a sample routine). However, treating cellulite is exactly like trying to lose weight or get very fit. You have to be determined to do it and to concentrate on incorporating other activities into your life which will also improve the appearance of your legs and thighs. The best results for treating cellulite with massage that I have seen were for someone who had ten treatments in the space of seven weeks (two half-hour cellulite massages a week for three weeks, then one massage a week for four weeks). As well as this, she halved the amount of caffeine and alcohol she drank each day, increased her plain water intake to 2.5 litres of water a day and did two hours of exercise a week (where she never did any exercise previously). She did not change her eating habits at all. In that time she managed to drop one dress size and showed significant improvement in the level of muscle tone on her legs, hips and thighs.

I know that massage of the abdomen will help to relieve my daughter's IBS, but she will not let me touch her abdomen. What should I do?
Irritable bowel is often identified by its symptoms of alternating constipation and diarrhoea. Those suffering with this condition frequently report that their bellies always feel tender, whether they are bloated with the constipation or have just experienced the diarrhoea. While massage will help to ease the spasms they experience and bring about more regular contractions in the bowel (and a more regular bowel habit), your daughter may find any pressure in this area painful unless she controls it herself. Your best bet is to explain how and why massage of the area will help, and encourage her to massage her own belly at least once a day. This will help to relieve any pain and discomfort she is experiencing and she will quickly see that it will not cause her pain for long. When you teach her to massage her belly for herself, emphasize the need to keep the movements slow and rhythmic. Later on, as she becomes more comfortable, you can introduce deeper movements (like petrissage) to help shift any faecal matter during times of prolonged constipation.

My friend has rheumatoid arthritis. Can massage offer pain relief?

Yes. Arthritis involves pain, stiffness and swelling of a joint. With rheumatoid arthritis this is an autoimmune condition (one where the body begins to attack itself) that often develops following a virus. If you choose to massage your friend, there are some special precautions you must both take. First, do not press hard. Your pressure should be lighter than normal, even if they are not in the middle of a flare-up (where the condition feels particularly bad). Second, work *around* but not *on* the affected joints. Third, keep your treatment short. Often someone with rheumatoid disease gets exhausted quickly when they receive a treatment. Your first treatment might only be 15 minutes long; you can increase the length of the treatment gradually if they are responding well. Fourth, make sure your friend is not involved in any major or unexpected activities after the treatment. Sometimes they can feel so well after a massage that they take advantage of the pain-free time to do something extreme – like a lot of gardening, perhaps – and this triggers a flare-up.

Will massage before a sports event help as a warm-up exercise?

Yes. Warm-up treatments are one of the key ways that sports massage therapists support their athletes prior to big events. It can be particularly useful if you know that an athlete either has an injury or is prone to injury in a particular area that cannot be effectively, quickly or easily warmed up. Massage will get right to the area of discomfort; and the massage therapist can also assess the muscles or joints in question and work out whether additional support or treatment is necessary. Massage can also help to improve motivation and performance if received regularly.

My partner has very high blood pressure. Would massage be dangerous?

High blood pressure is one of the conditions that is contraindicated for massage (see page 33). This does not mean that your partner cannot receive massage; quite the contrary – under certain conditions regular massage will help them to control and reduce their blood pressure. However, this is a condition that must be taken seriously. Check with their doctor that they are happy for you to massage your partner, and make sure your partner is taking any medications that have been prescribed (the massage will not take the place of medication). Assuming you have been given the all-clear to proceed, keep your movements slow and rhythmic; do not apply a lot of pressure, especially not at first. After a few treatments you may feel more confident about applying additional pressure, but this should never be to the point at which they find it painful. For best results, see if you can give them a very short massage twice a day (at the start and end of the day).

If massage affects blood sugar levels, how would it affect someone who has diabetes?

The answer depends on which type of diabetes the person has – insulin-dependent (they inject insulin several times a day in order to lower their blood sugar levels) or non-insulin-dependent (in which case they have to control their blood sugar levels by watching what they eat). Diabetes is also on the list of contraindications to massage, so you must be very careful when you treat someone who is diabetic (see page 30 for details of what to expect). Generally, massage will lower the blood sugar levels because it encourages the body cells to absorb sugar, thereby mimicking some of the actions of insulin. The most important thing to find out if you are massaging a diabetic is when they last ate and when they last gave themselves some insulin. Although we generally encourage people to have a massage on an empty stomach (or at least to wait a while after a meal before having a treatment), when massaging a diabetic it is a good idea to ensure that they ate recently and/or gave themselves a bit less insulin following their snack than they would normally do. Where it might be normal to offer someone a glass of water after a massage, a diabetic would benefit from some fruit juice or a biscuit instead.

Does massage have to be painful to be beneficial?

No. It is usually more beneficial when you are comfortable enough to relax, as one of the common reactions to pain is to contract your muscles. There are times, however, when the therapist does need to work a muscle quite hard in order to release any muscle fibres in spasm or reduce the size and appearance of trigger points (see page 111).

the benefits of massage

contraindications to massage

Contraindications exist where there are very good reasons to either avoid massage or proceed with extreme caution. Professional therapists tend to divide the contraindications into three main types:

- ❧ total contraindications – where massage should be avoided completely;

- ❧ local contraindications – where you avoid massage in certain areas;

- ❧ medical contraindications – where you should not massage unless you have the permission of the person's GP, or their specialist if they are receiving specialist medical care.

As with any situation of this type, there are sometimes grey areas where you might be able to proceed if you are very careful and *if* you know what you are doing and why. This chapter outlines the reasons behind the contraindications, to give you a deeper understanding of how and why massage therapists need to take additional precautions in certain situations. Remember, the general rule is that when you are uncertain (and perhaps you do not know what it is that the person is suffering from), it is best to avoid treating the person and suggest that they visit their doctor for clarification. It is also important to recognize when you are out of your depth and refer the person on to someone else. Working in ignorance is worse than not working at all.

Total contraindications

There are only a few situations where you must completely avoid doing a massage; when you take a look at the list, you will see that the reasons for avoiding a treatment are very sensible.

Any contagious or infectious skin condition

Where a contagious or infectious skin conditions exists (for instance, scabies), it is important to avoid treating the person with massage as you run the risk of cross-infection; not only could you spread the infection to another part of their body, but you could pick up the infection yourself and, potentially, pass it on to another person if you were to do another massage before you found out you had the infection and took the necessary precautions. Scabies is used here as an example because it is a particularly nasty infection (or infestation, as it involves tiny spider mites living under the skin) which is notoriously difficult to treat. If you were to contract scabies as a result of treating someone through massage, you would need to receive a special lotion from the chemist to treat your skin (and that of all the members of your household), and you would have to be very rigorous about boil-washing all towels, sheets and linens used in the household until the infestation had completely disappeared.

Other skin conditions which you may want to avoid include:

- impetigo
- ringworm
- warts
- verrucae
- athlete's foot

For conditions such as verrucae or athlete's foot, you can treat the rest of the body as long as you avoid the feet, specifically the infected area. In cases such as these, it is a good idea to put a plaster over the infected area to prevent any cross-infection as you work.

Severe, widespread psoriasis, eczema or dermatitis

Psoriasis, eczema and dermatitis are three fairly common and very uncomfortable skin conditions that all involve inflammation of the skin, along with other symptoms. Eczema is probably the most common, although there are a number of different types of eczema. Eczema means to 'boil over' in Latin, and involves redness, pain and itchiness, regardless of which type of eczema you have. Often eczema is linked to allergies (and sometimes appears alongside hay fever or asthma). Dermatitis means inflammation of the dermis (the deeper layer of the skin), and almost always occurs as a result of coming into contact with a substance that does not agree with you – for example, washing powders or household cleaners.

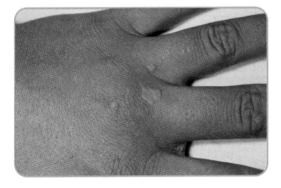

Warts are a contagious skin condition

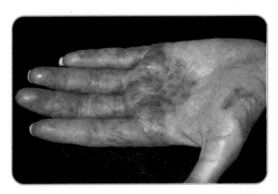

Dermatitis

Psoriasis, eczema and dermatitis are treated here as a separate category because there are times when massaging someone with these conditions is positively beneficial, as you can help the skin to return to a more balanced state if you work carefully and use vegetable oils. Times when it is beneficial to treat these conditions include when the person is between flare-ups or when they are aware that the condition is starting to get worse. It is particularly useful to treat these conditions if the person knows that the condition gets worse if they are under stress.

The important words in the heading above are 'severe' and 'widespread'. When these conditions are severe and widespread, the skin is very vulnerable, hypersensitive, extremely itchy and sometimes painful. Any new product or treatment introduced is likely to make the problem worse. Because the skin is damaged, raw and inflamed at these times, it is also far more prone to infection, so unless you are very careful about cleaning your hands before and after treatment with antibacterial cleansers, you will not be helping the situation at all.

Epilepsy

Epilepsy is a condition with which you must be extremely careful, especially if you do not know how to recognize if the person is having an epileptic episode. The short description of epilepsy is that the sufferer experiences sudden, unexpected electrical storms in the brain. There are two types of epileptic attack: petit mal and grand mal. When a petit mal occurs, the person appears to stop hearing or recognizing what they are doing, losing consciousness, but maintaining posture; this person may be accused of being a frequent daydreamer. Even more worrisome is when such symptoms progress to a grand mal – or

full seizure – which may involve uncontrolled muscle spasms and a loss of consciousness which can be frightening to watch if you are not familiar with first aid methods for treating epilepsy or if you have never seen a loved one experience a fit before.

Medical treatment for epilepsy involves specific drugs that must be taken regularly, especially if the person has frequent seizures. It cannot be emphasized enough that massage (and any other complementary therapy) cannot replace medical treatment for a condition like epilepsy. Nor is it appropriate to massage someone while they are having a seizure: not only would this be contrary to first aid procedures, but someone in the throes of a seizure could also fall off any couch and/or could hurt you in the process.

However, this does not mean that someone who is epileptic and taking medication regularly is never allowed to have a massage. This would be a good example of a situation where a massage therapist would ask for written permission from their epileptic client's doctor, stating that it was acceptable for them to receive massage. Please bear in mind that because of the severity of the condition, it is advisable that only a qualified massage therapist (who will usually have a first aid qualification as well) works with an epileptic client, and then only if they feel sufficiently confident to proceed.

Any untreated severe medical problem

Some untreated medical problems are obvious – a broken bone that has not been set or a case of whiplash where the person is still waiting to see a physiotherapist. But what about other, less apparent, problems? The quickest way to identify if something might be serious involves asking the following questions:

- ❧ Is there pain?
- ❧ Have you noticed any recent changes in sleep, bowel habits, weight or how you feel?
- ❧ Have you been prescribed any medications and are you taking them?
- ❧ Have you recently started taking/eating something new that might be making you feel different?

Please note that all these questions are deliberately designed to get the person to start making connections for themselves about how they are feeling. Massage therapists do not and cannot diagnose a condition, even if they might suspect that something is wrong. What they can do is recognize certain symptoms as being potentially dangerous and either suggest the person goes to the doctor or, if they feel very strongly about the situation, refuse to treat the person until they have seen a doctor and had the situation checked out.

Pregnancy during the first 16 weeks

Pregnancy is a wonderful time to receive massage treatments and many women who do so during their pregnancy report that it helps them to relax and feel more mobile as the pregnancy progresses, reducing oedema and relieving the sudden aches and pains that can occur at various stages in the pregnancy. Generally, it is considered wise to refrain from having massage for at least the first trimester (3 months or 12 weeks), and many therapists feel that it should be avoided for the first 16 weeks. During this period, the pregnancy is

at its most vulnerable – hormone levels are changing rapidly in order to maintain and stabilize the pregnancy and the foetus does not fully implant into the uterus until somewhere between weeks 8 and 12. Up to that point, a miscarriage is a very real possibility.

This does not mean that massage can bring on a miscarriage, but it is always wisest to let the body stabilize on its own until the first trimester is over, and then introduce massage as a means of supporting the ongoing pregnancy.

Any conditions being treated by a doctor or medical specialist without their written approval

Massage is a complementary therapy, which means that it works *alongside* other forms of treatment, such as conventional medicine, and does not replace them. Without detailed discussions with the person's doctor about what treatment they are receiving and what it is designed to do, you would not necessarily be aware of how massage might interfere with or potentially disrupt the treatment process. For instance, a massage might increase the effects – or certain side effects – of a particular medication, or it might mask some of the symptoms the doctor needs to know about to arrive at an accurate diagnosis.

Generally, massage is more likely to be seen by the doctor as a harmless addition to the support of most medical treatments, but if the person asking you to treat them is seeing the doctor regularly for something and/or is taking medication of any kind, you need to have permission from the doctor to work on them.

When under the influence of alcohol or recreational drugs

Massage stimulates the circulation and encourages body cells to absorb nutrients (and sugar) faster than usual; which means it will increase the effects of any substances. As it also increases the skin's ability to sweat effectively, increasing the release of water from the body, not only will you feel as if you have drunk more than you actually have, but the symptoms of a hangover (many of which relate to dehydration) will be stronger than usual.

Local contraindications

Bruises

Bruises occur where blood vessels (usually small capillaries) have been damaged and blood floods into the muscles, skin or underlying tissues, causing the familiar discoloration process to begin. Although people will often be seen rubbing the area after receiving the damage that will result in a bruise, massage over a bruised area is strongly discouraged, not only as it can prove painful, but also because it sometimes makes the bruising worse.

As bruises are a local contraindication, you can massage the person in other areas of the body, away from the bruise. However, it is always worth reminding someone that they have bruised a particular part of their body, especially if it looks large, as you will find that some people are not aware of having damaged themselves. Bruising, where it appears extensive, can sometimes be an indication of a more serious situation.

Cuts, grazes, open wounds, rashes, bites, stings, burns

Whenever the skin is damaged in some way, the use of any treatment involving a product (cream, oil or gel) and its application runs the risk of introducing some kind of infection. Cuts, grazes, burns and wounds need to be avoided, although you can work around the damaged area. With rashes, it is important to know what the rash is before you go anywhere near it (for instance, it could be something contagious, in which case you would need to avoid treating the person completely).

Where bites and stings are concerned, you will often see the body's natural immune response in play – an inflammation will usually appear around the affected area. This inflammation involves white blood cells that are hard at work to contain and destroy any invading pathogens (disease-causing substances) and any toxins injected by whatever stung the individual. Because massage increases blood circulation and reduces swelling, you could potentially disrupt the healing process, sending any toxins further afield, rather than having them contained and dealt with close to the site where they entered the body.

First three days of menstruation – deep abdominal massage

Deep abdominal massage needs to be avoided during the first three days of menstruation because it can increase the flow of menstrual blood. If the person who is being massaged tends to have very heavy periods anyway (this is called menorrhagia), this blood flow can be so excessive that they could experience some of the symptoms associated with shock from blood loss – nausea, dizziness, light-head-edness, feeling faint, actually fainting, feeling thirsty and weak, occasionally experiencing heart palpitations and a drop in blood pressure.

This does not mean that someone cannot receive massage at all during this time. Massage can actually help to reduce the effects of painful periods (dysmenorrhoea), but during the first three days, keep massage a bit lighter than usual over the abdomen (or possibly avoid abdominal massage altogether if you know the person tends to have very heavy periods) and concentrate your efforts in other areas where pain relief would be appreciated – the lower back, for example. If a person experiences a lot of pain, you can encourage them to massage their own abdomen in a slow circular movement (see pages 36 and 69) to relieve the pain. Make sure you warn them that this can increase blood

flow and that they should stop the massage if they feel uncomfortable. In practice, I have found that clients with painful periods who classed their menstrual flow as 'normal' (meaning a period lasted five days on average, with the first three days showing the heaviest flow) would note that while self-massage of the abdomen did relieve the pain effectively, they saw a great increase in the flow of blood on the first couple of days especially, and that when they performed the massage regularly during their period, the period was heavier, but shorter, often lasting only three days.

Deep abdominal massage during pregnancy

Although pregnancy was mentioned under total contraindications for the first trimester to 16 weeks, you can proceed with massage after this time. However, deep abdominal massage should be avoided during pregnancy for several reasons. First, you still have the enhanced blood circulation which caused concern during the first trimester and which is an ongoing concern if the pregnant woman has been experiencing any spotting (light blood flow, despite the pregnancy) or if the pregnancy is unstable. Second, deep abdominal massage can be uncomfortable for mother and baby if pressure is too great, especially as the pregnancy progresses. Third, as the baby gets larger, strong pressure either on the abdomen or the lower back (if the mother is seated and her belly is supported by a cushion or if she is leaning into a chair) can put pressure on the inferior vena cava (one of the main veins which takes blood from the body back to the heart), which can make the mother feel faint, nauseous, dizzy and weak. Fourth, remember that because massage can increase blood flow through the circulatory system, it is possible that it might lead to blood pressure alterations in the mother or bring on premature labour in unstable pregnancies. Massage is often used during labour itself to relieve pain and to encourage stronger, more effective contractions.

Immediately after a meal

A massage is not advisable straight after a meal as it can be very uncomfortable – particularly abdominal massage when your stomach is full. On a more physiological note, one of the things that happens to your body after a meal is that blood supply is increased to the abdominal area in order to effectively absorb nutrients from food once it enters the small intestine (think about how tired and sluggish you feel after a heavy meal, when you want to just sit still and do nothing while your body digests its food). If you have a massage at this point, your body experiences the massage as exercise and will stop the digestion/absorption process and shunt the blood to the skin and skeletal muscles instead. As a result, food remains uncomfortably in the system and any nutrients may not be absorbed effectively and efficiently.

Diarrhoea

While it is unlikely that anyone who has diarrhoea is actually going to want a massage, it is inadvisable to use abdominal massage at this time as you can make the diarrhoea worse. Please note that this contraindication is based on the assumption that the diarrhoea is part of a reaction to an intestinal bug or food poisoning and is not a regular occurrence. If your stools are always very loose, it is worth discussing this with your doctor or speaking to a nutritionist about making changes to your diet. If you experience diarrhoea regularly,

perhaps as a symptom of irritable bowel syndrome, you can receive massage without problems on the days when you are not experiencing diarrhoea.

Varicose veins

Varicose veins are caused by a malfunction of the semilunar valves in the veins. Blood tends to pool in the area and the veins become distended. While light pressure (effleurage) can be beneficial to encourage venous return, deep pressure and any vigorous movements should be avoided. The area can be worked on following surgery, but proceed with caution and wait until after the doctor or surgeon has given permission for massage to begin. Remember that varicose or even surface veins (where the veins appear close to the surface and where they might sometimes

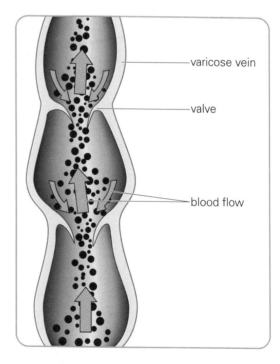

Varicose vein with an incompetent valve and reverted blood flow

be distended for a short period of time) can be painful to touch. Ask for regular feedback from the person receiving the massage, to ensure that they are not experiencing any pain.

Recent scar tissue

Recent scar tissue needs to be avoided in case the pressure of the massage causes the scar to open up or bleed. Scars tend to heal fastest at the skin's surface, with deeper tissues taking longer to heal. Healing tissue needs to be left alone as far as possible to heal on its own. With care, massage can begin to take place two to six months after the scar tissue is formed, with the length of time allowed based on the extent of the scarring and its location. When in doubt, ask the client for permission from their GP for massage to take place.

Over areas of inflammation, swelling or pain

Areas which are painful to touch and which are inflamed for no apparent reason should be avoided until medical advice is sought.

Medical contraindications

Medical contraindications generally refer to those conditions where you are not advised to treat the individual unless you have the permission of their doctor or specialist. As with anything else, there are certain situations where you could proceed with care as long as you understand what you are doing and why, and take special precautions.

Diabetes

Diabetes is a very important contraindication to bear in mind because of the physiological changes that can occur to someone who has had diabetes for some time, especially if they have not been careful about maintaining their blood sugar levels. The lack of care is more common in those who are non-insulin-dependent, who generally control their blood sugar levels through diet and exercise rather than by injecting insulin on a regular basis. However, both groups of diabetics need to be observed carefully before and during treatment because of the higher-than-average risk of the following symptoms:

- damaged nerve endings, which may be less sensitive to pain and could bruise easily if too much pressure is used;
- skin that is less flexible and elastic, often dry or damaged and may be easily cracked (diabetics are often advised to take particular care of their skin, using moisturizing products regularly and ensuring that they do not have very hot baths or showers);
- skin that heals more slowly (you should make them aware of any cuts or sores you notice, especially in areas they might not see themselves – feet, backs of legs or on the shoulders and back);
- a greater chance of infection, especially skin infections, such as athlete's foot or ringworm (so you run a higher chance of cross-infection);
- oedema;
- poor circulation.

Remember that one of the effects of massage is to lower blood sugar levels, so it is important to check that someone who is diabetic has eaten something shortly before beginning a massage, or that their blood sugar level is not at its lowest prior to treatment. It is useful to have fruit juice or a biscuit waiting for them after the treatment rather than a glass of water (as you might offer another client), just in case their blood sugar levels have dropped significantly during the session.

Heart conditions

The emphasis that massage places on circulation and the cardiovascular system cannot be underestimated. Treatments do affect blood pressure, raising it where massage is vigorous and involves deep abdominal massage, and generally lowering it where it is slow, rhythmic and soothing. Severe heart conditions must be taken into account if a change in blood pressure or circulation could affect the person's well-being.

Medications for a serious illness

While this contraindication suggests that you avoid treatment when receiving medication for a serious illness, it is worth discussing the potential effects of massage with your doctor where you are taking any medication, including antibiotics. For example, some antibiotics make the skin more sensitive to light, heat and other substances (which is one of the reasons you are told to avoid sunbeds or bright sunshine when on specific antibiotics). Massage does involve treating the skin and should therefore be carried out with additional care where it might affect the absorption of the medication or increase any

side effects. As mentioned in chapter 2, massage does increase the ability of the skin to absorb substances, so it will increase the absorption of any medications that are applied via the skin. This includes nicotine patches, HRT patches and/or any medicated creams or ointments.

Cancer

One of the key concerns with treating someone with cancer is the risk that you could encourage any cancer to metastasize (or move to another part of the body). This is particularly relevant as the most common way that cancer cells migrate is via the lymphatic system (or secondary circulation system). Massage is often used alongside cancer care, however, as it does help the individual to deal with the stress and emotional upheaval involved in facing cancer, as well as helping with some of the side effects of cancer treatment (including damaged skin, nausea, loss of appetite and a lowered immune response). It cannot be emphasized enough that you must have the written permission of the person's GP or oncologist if you are to massage someone with cancer who is undergoing radiotherapy or chemotherapy at the same time.

Post-operative

When someone has had an operation, they often remain officially in the care of their surgeon or specialist for some time after the operation, so that any unusual changes or circumstances can be noted and dealt with. While they are in the care of a medical professional, they are off limits to massage therapists unless there is written permission to treat. This contraindication relates not only to the length of time it can take for scars from surgery to heal, but also to the effects of any medications or painkillers the person might be taking during the recovery process.

Take as an example the scars that develop after surgery. Scars relating to ligaments (for instance, around the knee or ankle) might heal very quickly, but the ligaments themselves do not have as good a blood supply as other tissues in the body, so they are slower to heal. Leave them for a good four months before massaging in the area.

Abdominal scarring is also an area where you are advised to avoid pressure, as there will often be several layers of damaged organs that need to recover following surgery. Consider, for example, the advice often given to women who have had a Caesarian section: avoid driving for six weeks (the groin muscles are too damaged to allow the woman to make an effective emergency stop); avoid swimming and certain other types of exercise for two to three months (the effects on the underlying muscles apply again here, and there is risk of infection to the damaged uterus from immersion in chlorinated water); try not to get pregnant again for at least a year (because the healing process to all the tissues is not fully complete until then, so the muscles might not be able to stretch fully without tearing as the pregnancy progresses). This advice, usually given when a woman is discharged from the hospital, gives a clear indication of just how long it can take for the tissues in this area to heal completely. Gentle massage, particularly effleurage, would be beneficial and could occur two months after abdominal surgery, but this must be confirmed as acceptable by the doctor or surgeon. They may want to wait longer if the surgery took place in a different part of the body or if the condition being treated is very serious.

Severe swelling

Any swelling, especially if is in an unexpected place, should be dealt with or identified by a medical professional before you consider treating the individual with massage. Swelling can be the result of a number of things, some of which are potentially very dangerous to the person with the swelling. For example, it could be oedema, internal bleeding, a tumour, the result of a broken bone or a severe reaction to a bite or sting, as well as a number of less worrying possibilities.

Severe pain

Pain is a very good indication that something is wrong with the body. While massage can help with pain relief, it is usually advisable for the person to see the doctor straight away when they are in severe pain, as it will help the doctor to make an accurate diagnosis rather than have any symptoms either masked (or worsened) as a result of intervention by a massage therapist. Once an accurate diagnosis is made, it is possible the doctor might recommend massage if it will actively help the person's recovery from whatever is causing the pain.

Phlebitis or thrombosis

Thrombosis and phlebitis both refer to blood clots. In phlebitis you have inflammation of the blood vessels, usually the veins, which can sometimes lead to thrombosis. Thrombosis occurs where a blood clot within a damaged blood vessel breaks away and starts to move in the body. Deep-vein thrombosis, for example, occurs where such a clot appears in the legs and starts to move up the body towards the heart. Someone with a deep-vein thrombosis may experience pain on movement, but the more common symptoms are that one of their legs feels hard and swollen to the touch and may show a difference in skin temperature when compared to the other leg. The improvement in blood circulation can cause clots to break away or move faster than anticipated. Where these conditions are concerned, massage of any type should only take place with the written approval of the GP or consultant. Massage can help to lower high blood pressure (hypertension), but it is advisable to ensure that the GP or consultant is aware that the client is receiving regular massage, as this can sometimes affect the way in which the medication works (by increasing the rate at which it is absorbed by the body).

Sporting injuries

Sporting injuries are best left to the expertise of physiotherapists, osteopaths, surgeons (if relevant), chiropractors or sports massage therapists, as it is very important to treat the injury appropriately based on the severity of the damage and its location. While massage can be positively beneficial to the healing process, the depth of knowledge held by therapists who specialize in sporting injuries (or sports and remedial massage) should not be underestimated. This includes being able to recognize the severity of injuries as simple as a sprain or strain, knowing when it is safe to massage the injured area and exactly how long it should be left before proceeding with treatment.

contraindications to massage

casestudy: Saying 'no' to treatment

Sangita was in her fifties when she decided to try massage for the first time. Although she said initially that she wanted the treatment because of stress-related insomnia, when we started going through the consultation process together, a different picture emerged.

When you go for a professional massage treatment, you will go through an initial consultation process with your therapist. Sometimes this will involve you filling in a questionnaire (most of which is designed for the therapist to ensure that you do not have any contraindications to treatment). With other therapists you may sit down for as long as 20 minutes, discussing your health issues before commencing treatment. The questionnaire is designed to remind the therapist to get information about each of your body systems, especially where contraindications exist, so that they can provide you with a more detailed and personal treatment.

In Sangita's case, a number of the symptoms she described suggested that she really was not well enough to receive massage. She was experiencing blinding headaches; she knew her blood pressure was high, although she did not always take her medication for this (and had not taken it before coming to treatment); she was complaining of constant nausea, although she noticed she was eating less than usual; she also had pain and tingling running through her left arm. Taken together, these symptoms suggested that something could be seriously wrong with her cardiovascular system. While trying not to frighten her, I suggested that she visit her doctor as soon as possible, to ask if her symptoms could be checked out. When I spoke to her four days later, she told me that she had seen her doctor and, while her symptoms were investigated further, her medication had been changed and she had been advised by the doctor to look at ways of reducing stress in her life.

FAQs: About contraindications

Can I injure someone badly when I am massaging them?

If you pay attention to the contraindications (and do not treat someone if you feel uncertain about the situation), warm them up properly (with effleurage and plenty of kneading) before you do the more vigorous movements of the treatment (knuckling, petrissage, hacking, cupping, tapotement), you are less likely to cause damage. Do not forget to consider the individual requirements of the person receiving the treatment. Someone whose health is fragile – perhaps as a result of long illness, or because they are very elderly or very young – will not be able to take the same pressure as a fit adult, nor will they be able to comfortably enjoy a treatment of the same length. It is possible to make someone's condition worse if you do not know what you are doing or if you are too rough. Always ask for feedback, especially with respect to the pressure you are applying.

I have been an insulin-dependent diabetic for many years and have regular six-monthly check-ups at the hospital, but otherwise I am extremely healthy. Are you sure I need to have my doctor's permission to have a massage?

If your blood sugar level is stable then it is okay to proceed with the massage, but we have to be particularly careful of a number of things. First, make sure that you have eaten recently (as massage will lower your blood sugar level) and that you check your blood sugar level after the treatment. Second, because there are a number of side effects to diabetes (see page 30), we have to make sure that you give clear feedback about any pain or discomfort you feel during the treatment. We also have to make sure that you are aware of any cuts, wounds or abrasions (especially on your feet) you may have.

I have only had two glasses of wine at lunch before coming to have a massage. Are you sure I should avoid having a treatment? I feel nicely relaxed and this would complete my day.

One of the things that massage does is to improve the circulation of the body, getting nutrients to all body cells much faster than usual. When alcohol is involved, you will feel as if you have drunk much more (even as much as four to six glasses of wine), and you will probably experience the symptoms of a hangover. I would strongly advise you to avoid drinking alcohol before a treatment; if this is really impossible, then prior to treatment have a tall glass of water for each alcoholic drink and drink more water after the treatment as well. This should help you to avoid the worst of the symptoms.

Yes, I do have eczema all over my body, and yes it is very itchy, but the oil from the massage helps to relieve the itchiness. I really want to go ahead with the treatment.

With skin conditions like eczema, it is very important to avoid infecting the area and making the eczema worse. Generally, if the eczema is dry and neither cracked, bleeding or weeping, it is usually safe to proceed with the treatment. (The person giving the treatment needs to *thoroughly* cleanse their hands before and after working, and should avoid working on the skin when eczema involves open wounds of any description – some kind of infection would be almost certain and it is possible to pass any blood-borne diseases, such as HIV, to the therapist.) Given what you have said, I would suggest that you use the oil at home on a regular basis to soothe your skin and only have massage when you feel that your eczema is under control.

I have broken my collarbone, but why does that mean that I cannot have a back massage? I am sure it would relieve the pain and swelling.

One of the reasons we avoid massaging in the region of a broken bone is that the muscles around the bone usually go into spasm in order to keep the bone in one position while it is mending. As well as having muscles in spasm, you will have noticed that there is some swelling around your collarbone, as fluid will gather in the area in order to keep the bone stable and to ensure that there are nutrients available to speed up the healing process. While this seems like a good reason to avoid massaging the upper chest and shoulder areas – where your collarbone is located – we also have to avoid giving a back massage at this time, because any pressure applied to the back will affect the collarbone, especially as it is attached to the scapula (shoulder blade). Key muscles, such as the trapezius, are also attached to the collarbone and we do not want to interfere with their role in helping to heal the broken bone.

I am on the first day of my period and am experiencing a lot of pain, especially in my abdomen and lower back. I really want to have a massage. Can you help?

Massage, particularly deep abdominal massage, is contraindicated on the first three days of a menstrual period because it can increase the flow of blood at this time.

As a result, it is best avoided if you tend to bleed very heavily or if you occasionally feel faint from loss of blood in the first few days of your period. In other circumstances, gentle massage, particularly of the lower back, would probably be helpful. For best effects (and regardless of how much you bleed), you may want to consider self-massage of your abdomen instead. Simply massage your belly slowly and firmly in a clockwise direction, taking the movement low down between your hip bones. Heat can also help to reduce pain from cramping, so a hot water bottle, or the equivalent can help to reduce any pain experienced.

My baby has nappy rash, which I understand is a kind of dermatitis. Should I avoid massaging her?

In this particular case, I think you are safe to proceed with massaging her away from the area where she has the nappy rash. If the nappy rash is severe, you may want to think about what products you are using to cleanse and protect this area and whether you should change them. Check that you are keeping any jars or tubes properly sealed and that your hands are very clean both before and after changing a nappy. Check the extent of the rash to ensure that it is not the nappy itself (if using disposable nappies) or your detergents (if using terry nappies) that your baby is reacting to. You may want to speak to your GP or health visitor about the rash if it is slow to disappear. Sometimes nappy rash occurs as a baby is teething, or in nursing infants as a reaction to something the mother is eating. Otherwise it should disappear very quickly.

equipment and techniques

O ne of the most useful things you can
do to prepare for a massage is to care
properly for all the equipment you
need – that includes looking after yourself.
As a holistic form of treatment, massage
involves the body, mind, spirit and
environment of the person receiving the
treatment. Make your treatment the best
you can by considering these same aspects
for yourself: that you are using your body
(and weight) effectively as you work,
maintaining your posture; that you keep
your mind focused on the massage you are
giving; that you work when you are feeling
positive (if you are feeling low or
disinterested it will show in your treatment);
and that you make the environment in
which you are working as clear, coordinated
and coherent as your treatment.

massage equipment

The most important equipment you use when you are massaging someone is your own body. An effective massage therapist learns to use their body weight to the best advantage when carrying out a massage; they maintain good posture throughout the treatment and their hands, shoulders and forearms do not suffer overmuch as a result of the work they are doing. You need to take care of yourself and your physical health to maintain your effectiveness as a massage therapist – and this should be your foremost concern. However, there are a number of other items that are also significant in the process of carrying out a massage, and it is those items which we will concentrate on in this chapter.

Towels

Massage is generally a very demanding activity where towels are concerned. You will find that you get through towels very quickly as you really need a minimum of three clean large bath sheets per treatment, or two large bath sheets if you are using a massage couch with a towelling cover. Additional smaller towels are also very useful if you roll them up to form bolsters for knees, ankles or necks, or for added comfort around the face hole if you are using a massage couch.

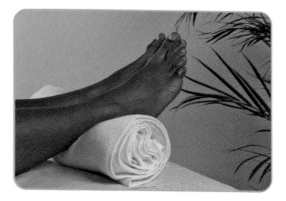

Making a bolster: Fold a hand towel in half lengthwise, then roll it tightly into a sausage shape. Use a piece of couch roll (if you have it) to wrap around the towel roll and tuck into the ends to maintain the shape of the roll and protect the towel from excess oil.

39

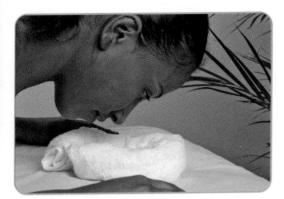

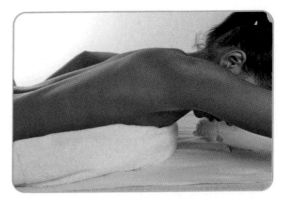

Making a face ring for a massage couch: Roll the short edge of a hand towel towards its middle, rolling up about one third of the towel. Place the rolled section on the top of the couch, around the edge of the face hole, and tuck the excess towel through the face hole, securing it in the base of the couch cover.

Making a long bolster: This is very useful if you have a client who either has large breasts or is very self-conscious about her chest area, as you can use it when she is lying face down on the couch to shield and/or support any tissue visible on the side of the body. Take a large bath sheet and roll it tightly along the length of the towel. Place the bolster on the couch so that the person being treated can rest their forehead on the middle of the bolster and the majority of the bolster will rest to either side of their body.

Towel management

Towel management is a term used to describe the discreet handling of towels so that only the body part you are working on is exposed during the treatment. Handling the towels properly will also keep the client warm and secure during the treatment. Every therapist has different ways of managing this carefully. My preferred method is shown below.

Getting the person onto the table

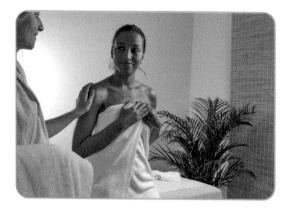

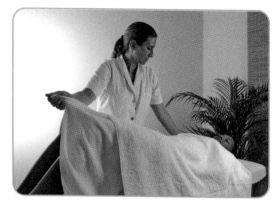

1 One large bath sheet is wrapped around them when they are undressed. Get them to sit on the table and lie back.

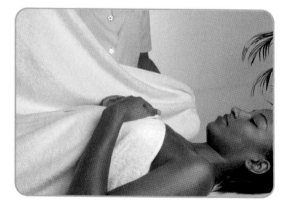

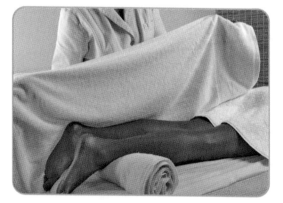

3 As the client lifts their hips, you grab hold of the towel they had wrapped around their body (now loosened), hold the upper towel in place and whip the lower towel out.

2 Cover them with another bath sheet, placed transversely across the body. Get them to loosen the towel they have wrapped around them.

4 Use the lower towel to cover the legs, placing it longitudinally along the lower body.

Exposing the legs

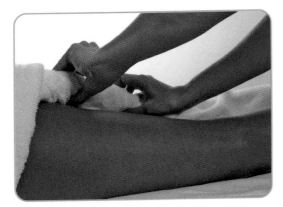

5 If you know you are going to be doing percussion movements, like hacking and cupping, you need to roll the towels very tightly to ensure that they do not move during the treatment. Roll the longitudinal towel under, and either fold the transverse towel back or roll it under and tuck it tightly against the person's body.

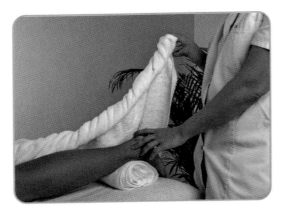

6 When you cover them up afterwards, take the edge of the rolled towel and let it roll over the leg to complete.

Exposing the arms

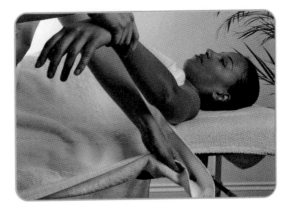

7 Leave the towel in place and just bring the arm out to work on top of the towel.

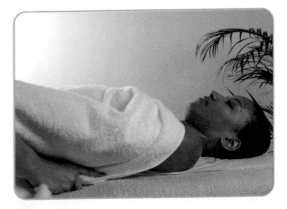

8 If the person needs warming up after the treatment, or if the couch seems too narrow, wrap their arm in the towel and tuck the end of the towel under their body to form a simple sling for the arm to lie in.

Exposing the neck and shoulders

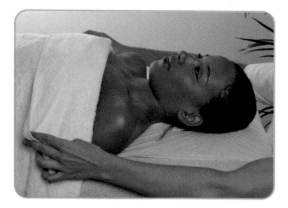

9 Fold the towel down, approximately level with the third rib.

Exposing the abdomen

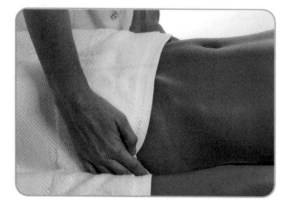

10 Ensure that the longitudinal towel comes high enough to cover any underwear and prevent it from being stained by the massage oil you are using. Fold this towel back evenly with the underwear. (Do not tuck it in the underwear.)

11 Fold the transverse towel up, usually in threes, until you have exposed the abdomen to the xiphoid process (the end of the sternum).

Rolling over

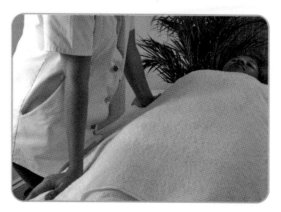

12 Hold the towels firmly down against the edge of the massage couch: one hand holds the transverse towel in place, the other holds the longitudinal towel in place.

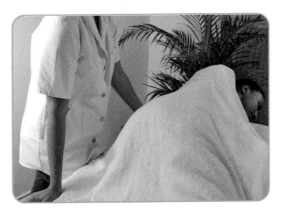

13 The client rolls away from you if they are lying face up, or towards you if they are lying face down.

Exposing the back and buttocks

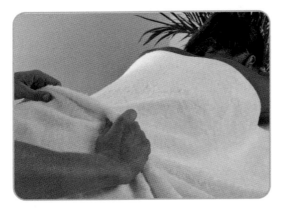

14 Run your hands over the towel until you feel the waist edge of the client's underwear.

15 Lift the edge of the underwear through the towel, adjust the waist downwards so that it is even with the gluteal fold, tucking a generous handful of towel into the underwear.

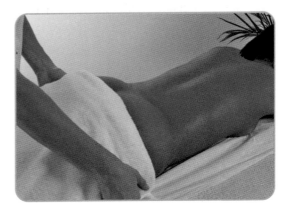

16 Fold back the towel to make a neat line across the body.

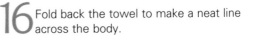

Pillows

For the most part, it is useful to encourage the person receiving treatment to lie on the couch without pillows, so that you have completely clear access to areas such as the neck while you are working. However, there are particular circumstances where pillows are definitely required for the comfort of the client. Examples include:

ঌ During pregnancy, when you may need to consider treating the person while they are lying on their side or in a partially seated position.

ॐ Any time that you treat someone in a partially seated position.

ॐ If someone has recently had breast implants, as it will be painful for them to lie face down.

ॐ If someone has a deeply curved lumbar spine and lower back pain. Try getting them to lie face down, with a pillow under their abdomen, as this will open up the area that needs additional work and can help to relax their muscles effectively during the treatment. They may also ask for a pillow under their knees or under their waist when they are lying face up. For the purposes of the treatment, it is advisable to encourage them to place the pillow under their knees if you are asked to give a preference.

ॐ If someone has a deeply curved thoracic spine. A very soft pillow folded in half lengthwise and placed between their shoulder blades and along their spine while they are lying face up on the table can help to stretch out specific muscles and improve posture.

Massage oils, creams and lotions

When Swedish massage techniques were first developed, the majority of massage therapists learned to massage with powders (including talc) as a lubricant to allow frictionless movement over the client's body. The therapist would apply powder to their own hands before working on the client's body. Today, powders are almost exclusively used by reflexologists (and even among reflexologists there is often a preference for cream or ointment as a lubricant rather than powder), while virtually all other body therapies have moved to using oils, creams, gels or lotions as a lubricant during treatment. Although powder would still allow for frictionless movement, it is the moisturizing and nutritive effects of the other substances on the skin which makes them more appealing to both clients and therapists.

If you look at the array of products available in any health-related shop, it can be quite difficult to choose a massage product that you will like and which will suit your needs. There are a number of issues to consider, including:

ॐ Cost: some pre-blended massage products, while beautifully fragranced, can be expensive. If cost is an issue, start by trying plain grapeseed or sunflower oil.

ॐ 'Slip': the thickness or viscosity of the oil accounts in part for how slippery it will make the skin and also how much of it you will need. Thicker, richer oils are sometimes worth having a small supply of, so that you can add a teaspoonful to another carrier oil to enrich it if the person you are treating has very dry skin. Two of the most useful rich oils are jojoba and avocado.

ॐ How quickly it degenerates: carrier oils, especially those of food quality, can go rancid if you do not take good care of them. They go rancid if they are kept under bright lights, if their lids are not properly fastened, if they are not kept at a stable temperature and, particularly, if they are kept somewhere warm. You can

Carrier oils and their features

Carrier oils	Features
Jojoba ****	Antibacterial, chemically similar to sebum (sebum will dissolve in jojoba). Use on all skin types, especially when sensitive, dry or dehydrated, or where eczema, acne or psoriasis exists. Can also be used to remove make-up.
Avocado ****	Anti-inflammatory, with some sunscreen properties. Use for eczema, dehydrated, mature and environmentally sensitive skin types. Use unrefined avocado oil by preference (a distinctive greenish colour).
Hazelnut ***	Mildly astringent, stimulates circulation. Use for oily, acne vulgaris or hormonally and stress-related sensitive skin. Avoid for acne rosacea.
Macadamia nut ****	As for jojoba, chemically similar to sebum. Good for dry and mature skin.
Peach kernel **	Pleasant fragrance, slightly richer than sweet almond, but with similar properties. Useful for normal, dry, dehydrated and sensitive skins.
Calendula ***	Anti-inflammatory, reduces scar tissue. Use for dehydrated, damaged or irritated skin. Very useful at helping to prevent and to repair stretch marks.
Sweet almond **	Use for chapped, inflamed or irritated skin, where eczema and dermatitis exist. Useful for normal or dry skin types.
Evening primrose *****	Helps to rebalance sebum secretions, mildly anti-inflammatory. Use for dry, oily or hormonally sensitive skin, as well as for acne, eczema and psoriasis. Generally sold in capsule form (simply pierce capsule and add to another carrier oil).

tell an oil is rancid not only by its characteristically stale smell, but also because it sometimes has a residue around the neck of the bottle. Bearing these features in mind, it is useful to keep your carrier oil in a cool, dark environment and to buy it in relatively small quantities if you are not using it regularly. On average you will use about 25–30 ml of carrier oil for a full body massage, which means that one litre will last for 32–40 treatments. Certain carrier oils, while useful, are quicker to degenerate than others. These include hazelnut, wheatgerm and corn oil. If properly cared for, most carrier oils will last for about six months.

How easily it is absorbed into the skin: lighter oils, such as grapeseed, sweet almond or peach kernel, will be absorbed into the skin very quickly, which makes these an ideal medium for massage if the person needs to get dressed in street clothes shortly after finishing the massage. Lotions and creams, while appearing to be even more absorbent than oil, tend to stay on the surface of the skin, although they do disappear quickly when used as part of a massage. If you choose to use a cream or lotion as part of a treatment, it is often advisable to use a thick, rich lotion as you will find the slip lasts for longer and you do not need to reapply cream during the treatment.

Carrier oils	Features
Coconut ✱✱✱	Relieves dry and itching skin. Use for dry, cracked, mature or environmentally sensitive skin. Monoï de Tahiti (a substance found in some baby skin care products) is made of gardenia flowers cold-pressed in coconut oil.
Apricot kernel ✱✱	Calms inflammation. Use for eczema and dermatitis, or for dry, mature and sensitive skin.
Grapeseed ✱	A very useful all-rounder for massage. Hypoallergenic, so a skin reaction to this oil is extremely rare. Usually costs less than most other carrier oils and can be purchased (along with sunflower oil) in large amounts in the supermarket.
Sunflower ✱	Useful for hormonally sensitive skin. An all-rounder.
Wheatgerm ✱✱✱	High in nutrients, moisturizing, cytophylactic. Good for dry or mature skin. Avoid use where there is a possibility of wheat intolerance or where skin is environmentally sensitive.
Argan ✱✱✱✱✱	Fantastic oil for use on the face, has a well-deserved reputation for preserving and healing skin, reducing the appearance of wrinkles, moisturizing and nourishing. Difficult to find in its natural state (you need to go to a wholesaler).

Price rating: expensive ✱✱✱✱✱, above average ✱✱✱✱, average ✱✱✱, below average ✱✱, cheap ✱ (all prices relative to carrier oils, not to other massage products)

Antiseptic wipes

It is useful to have antiseptic wipes to hand when carrying out a massage. Many therapists use these initially to clean their client's feet and, occasionally, hands before a treatment. As well as clearing the feet of any debris, it allows the therapist a chance to check the feet for any small infections, cuts or abrasions that might exist, in a place many people choose to ignore (and which is particularly relevant as a place of potential injury to diabetic clients). If necessary, the wipes are also invaluable for removing any excess oil from the feet prior to getting off the table (and thereby reducing the risk of slipping and falling after the treatment).

Plasters

Plasters are particularly useful if you need to cover up any small cuts or if you find small warts, verrucae or some athlete's foot on the client's feet or hands. Covering up the areas with a protective layer such as a plaster makes it possible for you to proceed with the treatment while not putting either yourself or the person receiving the massage at risk of cross-infection.

Protective clothing

The decision about whether or not to wear protective clothing or a uniform will depend on the individual and how they intend to practise massage. Certainly some form of uniform is expected when you take professional examinations in massage therapy. There are a number of benefits to wearing protective clothing when working in massage. First, whoever you are treating will get used to you always appearing dressed in a similar style; this adds a degree of professionalism to your treatment. Second, it means that only one item of clothing – the tunic top – runs the risk of being damaged by the oils you are working with, so there is less wear and tear on the rest of your clothing. Third, the tunic tops are designed for this style of use, so they tend to be made of a hard-wearing cotton blend, which can withstand the necessarily high temperatures of wash cycles required if the oil stains are going to be effectively removed after each wear.

When you are choosing a tunic top for massage, there are a number of essential features to look for:

ॐ predominantly cotton so that it will withstand a hot wash;

ॐ short sleeves (above the elbow) so that you can work with your forearms or elbows if required;

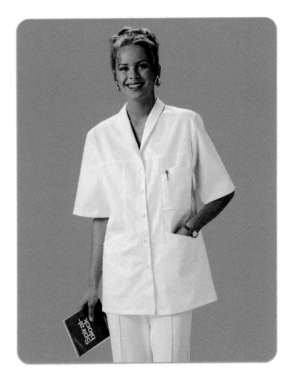

Protective clothing gives a professional image

ॐ stretchy or loose-fitting across the shoulders so that you are not limited in your movements;

ॐ not overly tight-fitting or suggestive.

Massage couch

A massage couch is the single most expensive item that anyone seeking to practise massage will purchase. Unless you intend to go on to train as a professional massage therapist, it is probably not worth the expense of investing in a couch. At the time of going to press, the cheapest couches available in the UK start at £125 +VAT and range upwards to £750 +VAT for particularly lightweight ones (or above this price for electric or hydraulic couches).

Choosing a couch is a big commitment to a potential career or a very serious hobby and, given the expense, it is worth thinking very carefully about what your intentions are for the long term. If you intend to go on to learn another discipline, you may need the couch to have additional features. If you intend to practise reflexology using the couch as a base, you would need to be able to extend the legs of the couch and raise its back so your client can be semi-reclined while receiving treatment and you can sit comfortably at the base of the couch with their feet at exactly the right height. If you want to train as a professional therapist and intend to travel with your couch to do home visits, you may be advised to look for the lightest couch you can find (these cost significantly more).

If you decide to go ahead with purchasing a couch, you can save a certain amount of money by opting to buy a couch that does not have adjustable height legs. This is advisable only if you intend to practise only holistic massage, reiki or aromatherapy, and will not be taking up any additional treatments (even sports massage would benefit from adjustable height legs, as you can lower the couch if you need to put more of your body weight into the treatment). You can identify the correct height for your couch by standing alongside the couch and making a light fist with your hands. At the correct height, your knuckles should just lightly rest on the couch.

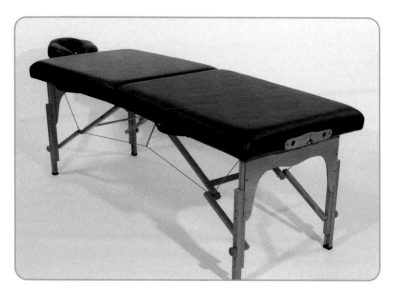

Couch roll

Couch roll, the paper roll that is used by professional therapists to cover the couch is an optional piece of equipment. It is used for hygiene purposes, especially if the therapist is using the same couch cover for more than one client. Some therapists choose not to use couch roll as it does not always feel nice against the skin. In these cases they are adding to their laundry bills accordingly. Couch roll is very easy to obtain, either through beauty and hairdressing suppliers or by mail order.

FAQs: About massage equipment

How do I get the smell of vegetable oil out of my towels? I have ruined several towels in the process of learning to massage.

This is a perennial problem for massage therapists and there is only one answer which I have found to work: wash the towels as soon as possible after use at the highest temperature your washing machine allows (usually 90 degrees) and use a liquid biological washing detergent. If you have experienced some delay before washing, or if the towels are badly stained, you can try soaking them first in a product that is designed to remove biological stains from baby clothes and nappies. Generally, I would recommend that you keep sets of towels specifically for massage and plan to replace them every two years if you are using them extensively.

Do I really need to use vegetable oil? Would baby oil do instead? Or how about something cheap, like corn oil from the supermarket?

I like to recommend vegetable oil as the carrier oil of choice because it is full of essential fatty acids and other vitamins which help to improve the health of the skin. If all you are worried about is getting enough slip in the massage so that your hands glide over the body appropriately, then baby oil is fine. Please remember that baby oil is petroleum-based and just acts as a barrier to the skin; it does not really absorb into the body effectively. Furthermore, anyone with very dry or sensitive skin might respond better to a vegetable oil (try grapeseed if they are hypersensitive). As for corn oil, yes, it is cheap, but it also tends to go rancid very quickly. Even olive oil, despite its strong smell, would be preferable. Grapeseed is also readily available in the supermarket and is not too expensive.

I sweat a lot and I am worried I might sweat so much during a treatment that it drips onto the person I am working on. What do you suggest I do?

This is something you need to address properly; if your sweat does fall onto the client, that is a serious breach of the acceptable hygiene that therapists need to observe. First, make sure there is adequate ventilation and airflow where you are working, so that you are less likely to sweat excessively. If ventilation means that the client feels cold, you can always cover them with extra blankets or a duvet while you work. Second, you must make sure that you take particular care over your personal hygiene immediately prior to starting a treatment, as sweat can give off a very distinctive odour. Third, you could try having a hand towel nearby and using it to blot your face, neck and hands while you are working. If you do choose to use the face towel, make sure that you place it in such a way that you can pick it up without touching the sweat with your hands. (If this were to happen, you would need wash your hands before continuing the treatment.)

My friend has breast implants and says that she finds it painful to lie on her stomach for a treatment. What do you suggest I do?

This is actually quite common and will also affect women who are breastfeeding (if their breasts are engorged) and those who have painful breasts as part of their premenstrual symptoms. You can try massaging them lying on their side, although this is not ideal if you want to do a good treatment for the back and shoulders. Try using two pillows – one to go above the breast area (so the head and shoulders rest on this) and one to go below the breast area (for the abdomen and hips). This will help to take the weight off the breasts and will ensure that they are not completely squashed when you are working.

Do I have to buy a massage couch? Can I practise without it?

Of course you can still do massage without a couch! Try working on the floor, as the person needs to be lying on a hard, flat surface for best effect – a bed would be too soft. If you are planning on practising professionally or taking professional examinations in massage, it is advisable that you buy (or borrow) a couch to practise on at home. If your intention is to work only in a salon, health centre or similar venue, where a couch will be provided, then it does not make sense for you to purchase a couch, except for short-term use while you are training. Do not spend too much money.

massage movements

Therapeutic and holistic massage is based on the use of a range of movements. Different therapists will class these movements in a variety of ways. I have found the simplest way to describe the groups of movements is as follows:

- effleurage: flowing, stroking movements;

- petrissage: grinding compression movements;

- percussion or tapotement: fast, tapping or beating movements;

- vibrations: quick, fluttering movements.

These movements are combined in sequences designed to encourage a return to optimum health.

Effleurage

Translated from the French, effleurage means 'flowing' or 'stroking'. Effleurage is used to start and finish any massage routine, as well as providing a means of linking other movements together or moving from one section of the body to another. Generally, such movements involve the whole palmar surface of the hand, with the hands relaxed and soft – the fingers usually closed, but flexing to follow the shape of the area being treated, rather than remaining stiff. When you are doing effleurage, you can vary the pressure of the movement – start very light, but get progressively firmer as the person gets used to your touch. A very effective effleurage will show the skin rippling ahead of your hands as you work. As you finish a treatment, your effleurage movements can get progressively lighter as a way of 'saying goodbye' to the body you are treating.

Effleurage also gives you an opportunity to assess any areas of tension, to identify places where the skin is either hot or cold to the touch and to plan how you are going to proceed with your treatment. Effleurage is also very useful to reduce lymphatic congestion or water retention, which makes it ideal as an intermediate stroke to repeat after deeper strokes, in order to encourage the removal of toxins from the muscles being treated.

Varieties of effleurage

Hands opposing

Turn your wrists so that the fingers of both hands are pointing towards each other.

Hand leading hand

The wrist of one hand rests against the membrane separating the index finger and thumb of the other hand.

Thousand hands

A faster version of effleurage, where you run the hands quickly along the area you are working on in order to warm the person up.

Standard

With your wrists straight and the fingers pointing in the direction of travel.

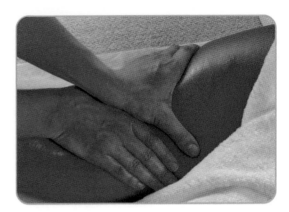

Hand leading hand

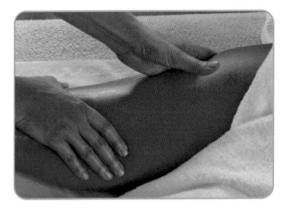

Thousand hands

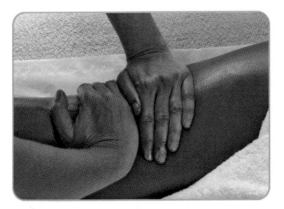

Hands opposing

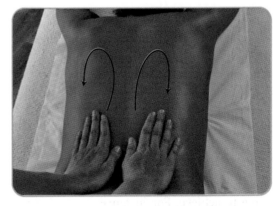

Standard

Back and forth

Usually done to the neck when the client is lying face upwards, with your fingers closed, moving your hands from the wrists as if they are windscreen wipers.

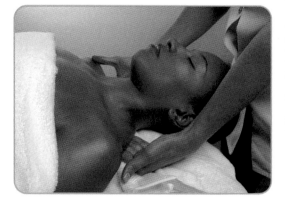

Back and forth

Petrissage

Petrissage encompasses a range of compression movements in which muscle or skin is compressed or ground against underlying bones or tissues. Regardless of which form of petrissage is being used, the movements are done with a smooth and firm pressure which is applied and then released. For example, petrissage with your thumbs tends to involve rotations over small areas of muscle, which means that the pressure remains firm as you take your thumb over and then off the area which is contracted.

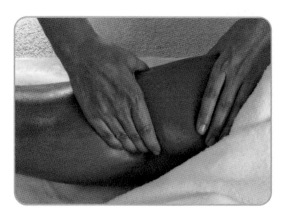

Kneading

Varieties of petrissage

Kneading

This movement is carried out as if you were kneading bread – flesh is picked up in one hand and then transferred towards the other hand with a back-and-forth movement. The speed and rhythm with which you do this movement allows for variety in what you are trying to achieve. For instance, a fast rhythm will be more effective at warming up the muscles and energizing the individual, helping them to feel more alert. A slow, smooth rhythm will help someone to calm down after a stressful day and will improve sleep. Kneading is designed to break down deep muscle tension and release any adhesions between the skin and the underlying muscles. It is also very useful for improving muscle tone and warming up the muscles prior to any sporting event.

55

Finger frictions

Frictions tend to be small circular movements over small areas, between the metatarsals or the metacarpals, for example. They are very effective at encouraging any waste products of metabolism (or any water retention) to return to the cardiovascular system and move from there to the kidneys for removal from the body. Finger frictions are also very useful if you need to work across muscle fibres when a muscle is very tight, painful or in spasm. Try finger frictions over the erector spinae, or if you find any particular areas of tension in the lumbar region of the back or around bony areas such as the knees, scapula, ankles, wrists or elbows.

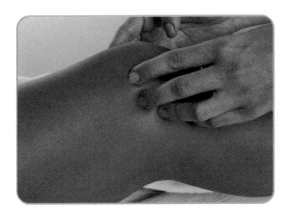

Finger frictions

Wringing

Wringing initially appears similar to kneading, although the movement is slower and involves more of a squeezing movement to the tissues. This is particularly effective over the gluteals or the lumbar region, as it combines the effects of a deep petrissage style of movement with a simple stretch to the area.

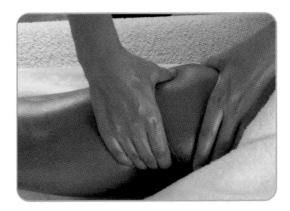

Wringing

Thumb petrissage

Similar to finger frictions, but this is done with the thumbs, which move in small controlled circles over areas of tension. This is particularly useful over the erector spinae, all the upper trapezius and neck muscles (both in the prone and supine positions) and around the scapula. Thumb petrissage is also a very effective tool in facial massage routines.

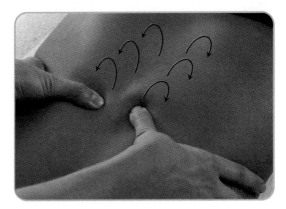

Thumb petrissage

Knuckling

This is carried out with the first and second phalanges of the fingers. Keeping your wrists straight in order to maintain pressure appropriately, the movement is a rotation from the wrist (but the fingers remain still). While you will see different varieties of knuckling, working with the wrists straight and the fingers still helps to ensure that any pressure applied will not damage the therapist's hands. This makes knuckling one of the more useful strokes if you find your hands and wrists are starting to hurt as a result of giving too many massages.

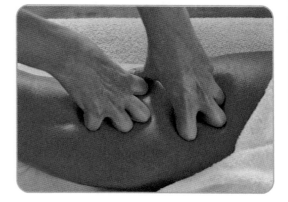

Knuckling

Percussion

Percussion, or tapotement, movements are the most stimulating and invigorating movements in the repertoire of a therapeutic massage therapist. The movements require a great deal of flexibility in the hands and wrists, as well as being rhythmic and fast. Student therapists often find these the hardest movements to learn, as doing them well (and making the appropriate sound when you are working) takes a great deal of practice and control.

Varieties of percussion

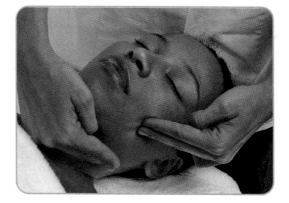

Tapotement

Tapotement

Originally, the term 'tapotement' was used to refer to a very light percussive movement on delicate areas such as the face and neck, or where a great deal of pain is present. To use tapotement in these areas, you might only use the fingertips in a circular, lifting movement.

Cupping

Making a loose cup shape with the hands, vigorous cupping movements are used on the body. For the most part, this tends to be particularly effective over the thigh area (and is essential as part of a treatment for cellulite or to improve muscle tone in this area). If the cupping is effective, you will quickly see a reddening to the area as blood is brought to the surface of the skin. This is because the

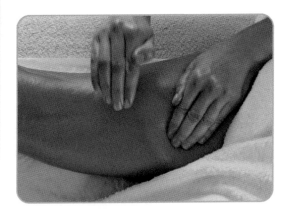

Cupping

cupping creates a miniature vacuum effect to pull blood to the area. When cupping is done correctly, it sounds like horses' hooves on a pavement. If the cup made by your hands is not deep enough, it will feel as if you are slapping the person you are working on.

Hacking

Using the lateral side of the fingers of each hand to hit the client in a rhythmic movement. This needs to be done very quickly to get the maximum effect and should be done over the whole of the area that you are working on. Keep your wrists loose and make sure that only the fingers hit the client, not the side of the

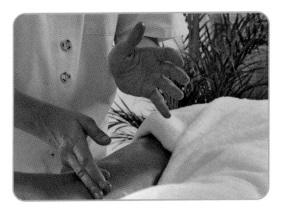

Hacking

hand (this will be painful to you and to the person you are treating).

Pounding

Make a light fist and use the side of the fists in a rotary movement to provide a gentle 'lifting' effect. This is very useful at the tops of the legs and over the gluteus maximus to help tone this area.

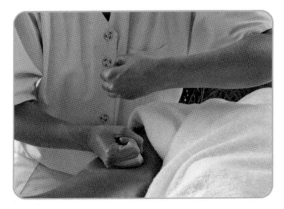

Pounding

Beating

Make a light fist and use the lateral side of the fist to gently hit the client over the large muscles of the body. This is best avoided in

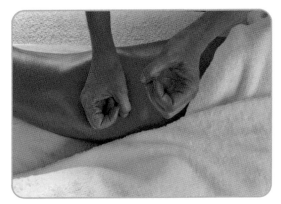

Beating

frail clients, but is very effective where the client has excellent muscle tone. Try using this over the calves, hamstrings and gluteals for best effect.

Hacking 'du poing'

Meaning 'with the fist', this is hacking done with your fingers curled. It is a deep movement and particularly useful where muscle pain and tension has been present for a long time.

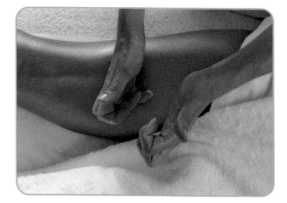

Hacking 'du poing'

Vibrations

These very gentle movements tend to be overlooked, but are invaluable if someone is suffering from nerve pain or is experiencing a great deal of tension. The gentle, trembling movements are done with thumb, fingers or the hand to specific tissues, usually over a particular nerve path to encourage deep relaxation.

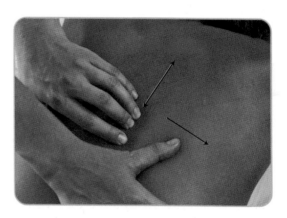

Vibrations

FAQs: about massage movements

I cannot seem to do hacking for more than about ten seconds without it starting to hurt me. What am I doing wrong?

This is a common problem, usually because you will be keeping your wrists and hands very rigid, instead of relaxing into the movement. Your hands should be loose and floppy, with most of the movement taking place in the wrist. People often find hacking difficult if they forget to breathe while they are working or if they bring their elbows in hard to their sides as they tense up during the movement. Keep your breathing regular and try sticking your elbows out more as you work. Although this looks funny initially, it will help you to relax while you practise the movement and it will not be long before you can do the movement easily and in comfort.

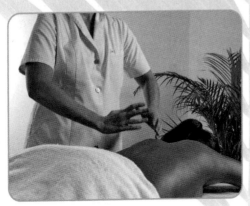

'Elbows out' with hacking

When I try hacking, my friends always say it hurts them. What should I do differently?

Most likely you are allowing the whole of the side of your hand to connect with the person you are massaging. With hacking, you should only allow your fingers to connect with their body. If you are hacking in the shoulder or neck area, this should only be the fingertips.

When I try cupping, my friends tell me it feels as if I am slapping them. What am I doing wrong?

You have not made a deep enough cup shape with your hands. When you practise, try bringing your thumb further down the side of your fingers, so that it is resting against the first knuckle of your index finger. Listen to the noise you make; when it is done properly, cupping should sound like horses' hooves on a pavement.

I find every time I do petrissage my thumbs start to hurt. How can I give an effective treatment without this hurting me?

There are a large number of different types of petrissage that you can use. Try reinforcing your thumbs (put one thumb over the other to press deeper, while still protecting your thumb), switching to knuckling or, when you feel very confident, working with your forearms or elbows instead – this will give you the deep pressure that petrissage is designed to achieve.

What should I do if I forget the next movement in the sequence?

Effleurage until you either remember the next movement in the sequence or become aware of an area that seems particularly tight or problematic, and then you can switch to more detailed work (kneading or petrissage) on that area.

Vibrations seem really lightweight – I am not putting any pressure into the movement. Does it actually do anything?

Yes, it does. Vibrations help to release any adhesions between the muscle and the overlying skin. When done properly, they are extremely relaxing to the client and help to finish off the treatment.

massage as a
holistic treatment

Massage is sometimes referred to as a holistic treatment – one which takes into consideration the physical, mental, spiritual and environmental circumstances of the person receiving the treatment. In practice, this means that the treatment you give should be different for each person. Learning a routine is a great way of getting started in massage, as it gives you a chance to practise all the different massage movements and to learn to massage someone with confidence. It is useful for you to think of the different massage movements as a set of tools, not as parts of a routine. Once you feel confident with the tools you are learning to use, you can begin to branch out and develop your own routine, using the movements to give more effective treatments, as you start to take into consideration exactly what the person receiving the massage needs in order to feel better.

As you get more experienced with massage you will find that you start to notice more when you are treating someone: you might become aware of temperature changes in different parts of their body; you will be able to tell the difference between a muscle in spasm and inflammation; and you will be able to see when a muscle has been tight for a long time and is starting to cause postural problems. As you start to notice these things, you will be that much more confident with the movements you are familiar with, which will allow you to branch out and adapt your treatment to suit the needs of the individual you are treating – perhaps working more over the lumbar and sacral region if this is where pain is more intense or frequent.

For the most part, it really does not matter which order you do the movements in. However, the routines suggested in this book, and those you will pick up in any massage class, are based on fundamental principles, all of which are designed to make the massage feel good for the client and which involve the minimum effort from the therapist for the maximum result. Start by assessing the person, warming up their muscles to encourage relaxation (effleurage); gradually introduce increasingly deeper strokes once they are

61

relaxed enough to take the extra pressure (kneading, knuckling, hacking, cupping); then gradually lighten your strokes towards the end of the treatment (effleurage and vibrations). Never do deep stretches on muscles which are not warmed up properly. The client will not have the necessary mobility at this stage and you could seriously hurt the muscles if they are in spasm and forced to stretch prematurely.

Client care, client modesty and client confidentiality

Professional massage therapists are expected to put their client's needs at the centre of the treatment and to recognize that there is more to a massage than the ability to exhibit the correct strokes and carry out a prescribed routine within the time available. To make your treatment truly client-centred, you should keep in mind the three concepts of client care, modesty and confidentiality.

Client care

This involves the practical steps you take to care for the client's well-being before, during and after the treatment. Appropriate care for the person you are massaging involves considering all their needs relating to the massage. If they are frail or find it difficult to move easily, you may need to help them on and off the surface you are treating them on. You will need to prepare appropriately for their treatment – have the treatment space ready and waiting when they arrive; ensure you have a calm, clean atmosphere in which to work; check they are comfortable and that the pressure you are applying is acceptable; avoid being interrupted; maintain strict hygiene; make sure your skills are appropriate for the person you are treating (and refer them on to someone more skilled if necessary); focus on the person you are treating for the duration of the massage.

Client modesty

The client's modesty and privacy must be respected at all times during and after the treatment. Removing their clothes will make most people feel very vulnerable (as well as making them prone to feeling cold). Remember only to expose the body part you are currently treating. If you have to leave the person for some reason, make sure they are properly covered before you depart. You also need to ensure that the person has privacy in which to undress and that they will not be observed as they are changing. Any notes you keep about the treatment must be locked up securely afterwards; any consultation you carry out must be done where no one can overhear it. Furthermore, it is expected that you will not pass judgement on anything they say, nor discuss it with anyone else.

Client confidentiality

Anything the person receiving treatment says during the treatment must be regarded as being in the strictest confidence and should not be discussed outside the treatment room. Similarly, any comments you have about their health or their body are not for discussion with anyone else. Occasionally you might need to discuss progress with another therapist if you need advice on how to proceed, but it should be understood that this discussion is in confidence and that the other therapist can maintain that confidentiality. If you are going to discuss the situation with someone else, you will need to have your client's permission to do so.

Hygiene

The role of hygiene in a massage treatment is extremely important. This relates not only to the room in which you are working, but also to the use of antiseptic wipes, couch roll and clean towels. Your personal hygiene is also important; massage is about nurturing and caring for the individual. How is someone going to judge your treatment if they suspect that you are unable or unwilling to nurture yourself? Things to pay particular attention to include ensuring you have very clean hands and nails, that you have recently bathed, that your breath is fresh, that you do not have any noticeable body odour and that you are wearing clean clothes and any long hair is tied back.

massage as a holistic treatment

effleurage massage

Effleurage is often the first stroke that you will learn when you start your massage course. Sometimes people can take it for granted as it seems so light, even if you are learning to put more pressure into the movements as you are working. However, it is extremely useful and, no matter how interesting or challenging the other strokes might seem to you as the practitioner, it is worth taking the time to experiment with carrying out treatments using effleurage alone. Effleurage helps to soothe and relax anyone you work on; it will warm them up and help to get the circulation going, as well as helping to disperse any oedema.

A treatment that only involves effleurage is indicated when you are working with someone who is in poor health, is very frail or very young. Newborn infants, for instance, respond to it very well, as do those with immune-related disorders, or where someone is recovering from a long-term and debilitating illness. It is also a very useful stroke to learn in order to help yourself – for instance, the effleurage routine for the abdomen is ideal as a means of support for women with painful periods, to prevent stretch marks during pregnancy and as a self-help method for people with irritable bowel syndrome (IBS).

Full body effleurage routine

Legs

1 Expose the right leg, apply oil over the entire leg.

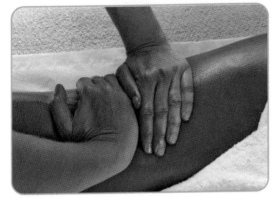

2 Hands-opposing effleurage over entire leg.

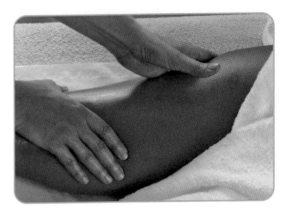

4 Thousand-hands effleurage over entire leg. Bring hands up over thigh, glide down the outside of the leg to ankle and repeat.

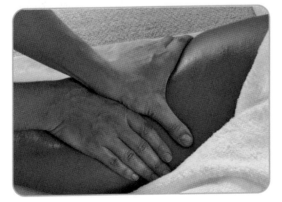

3 Hand-leading-hand effleurage over entire leg. Hands move up leg and thigh, glide down outside of thigh.

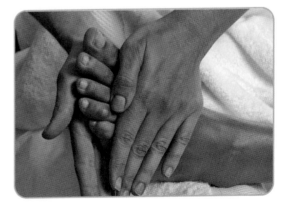

5 Vertical effleurage of the foot. Hands sandwich foot and move from toes to ankle, glide back up foot and repeat. Pressure is on the downward strokes, no pressure towards toes on return.

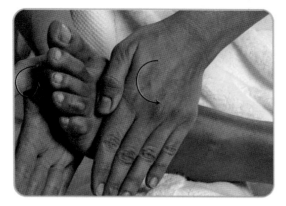

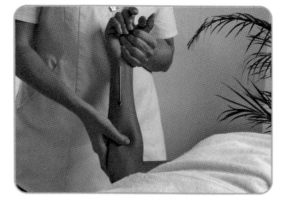

6 Rotary effleurage of the foot using fist into plantar surface. Hands rotate like train wheels.

7 Reflex strokes to finish. Repeat for other leg.

Arms

8 Expose arm, applying oil over entire arm and shoulder.

9 Effleurage over entire arm: one hand works up the medial side of the arm, over the shoulder and then down the lateral side of the arm; second hand holds the wrist to make sure the arm stays still.

10 Drainage to forearm: raise wrist, so you can drain down to the crease of the elbow (cubital crease) – drainage is done as if you are squeezing toothpaste out of a tube. Keep your hands quite firm, but the movement is not painful.

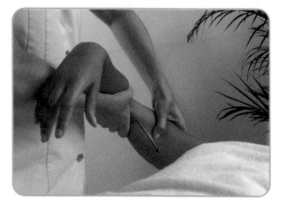

11 Drainage to upper arm: raise arm from the elbow (you hold the elbow so the arm can rest over your forearm) – movement is lighter and moves towards the armpit. Some people find the area between the body of the bicep muscle and the armpit quite sensitive, so keep pressure lighter.

67

massage in essence

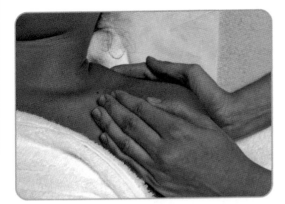

12 Double-handed drainage around the shoulder. Move hands back and forth in a sawing movement.

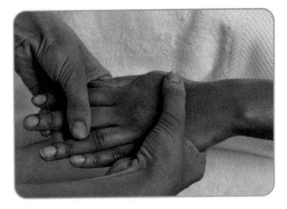

14 Vertical effleurage of the hand.

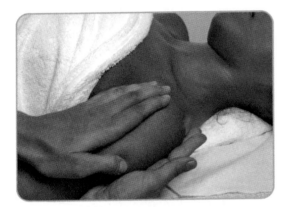

13 Squeeze and press down, stretching the muscles from the back of the neck (trapezius) and the upper pectorals – stretch to go all the way down the arm to the fingers.

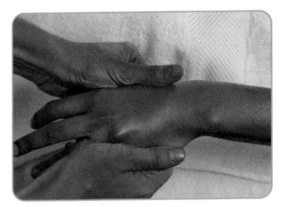
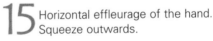

15 Horizontal effleurage of the hand. Squeeze outwards.

16 Reflex strokes to finish. Repeat for other arm.

Neck and shoulders

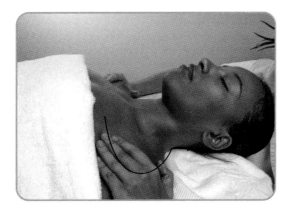

17 Effleurage over upper pectoral muscles, upper trapezius, deltoids and back of the neck. Start with your fingers meeting at the sternum, swoop your hands outwards over the shoulders, then round the back of the shoulders and up the back of the neck to the hairline. Bring your hands forward to the shoulders (do not squeeze or press on the sides of the neck) and back to the starting point.

18 Back-and-forth effleurage of trapezius: wrists move back and forth so hands cover the trapezius up to the acromion process and back again.

19 Thousand-hand effleurage to one side of the neck, then the other.

20 Repeat effleurage to both sides of the neck.

Abdomen

21 Expose abdomen, as you are standing to the person's right-hand side.

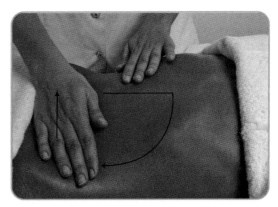

22 Circular effleurage: your left hand makes a circle, taking in as much of the abdomen as is exposed. Your right hand draws a straight line from the opposite hip to the hip closest to you.

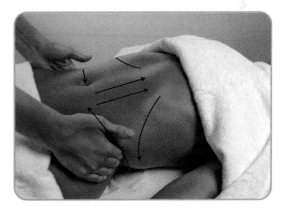

23 Lateralizing effleurage: start with your fingers at the person's navel, go upwards towards the xiphoid process, follow the line of the ribs around to the sides of the body (taking your hands as far under their waist as you can comfortably go) and lean back; as you straighten your back, your hands will help to stretch out the latissimus dorsi and external obliques, on the back and sides of the body.

69

24 Repeat circular effleurage to finish.

Legs – prone (face down)

25 Hands-opposing effleurage over entire leg.

26 Hand-leading-hand effleurage over entire leg.

27 Thousand-hands effleurage over entire leg.

28 Reflex strokes to finish. Repeat for other leg.

Back

29 Standing to the person's left side, expose the back and upper buttocks (down to the gluteal fold) and apply oil.

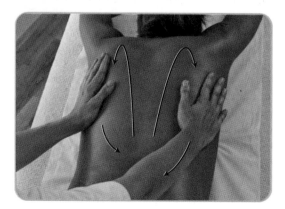

30 Standard effleurage up the back, along the erector spinae muscles, from the sacrum to the top of the shoulders, returning along the sides of the body (do not press as hard on the return).

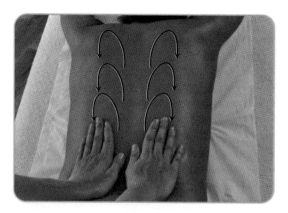

31 Fountain effleurage: three circles over the lumbar region and gluteus medius; three circles over the thoracic region; three circles over the upper trapezius and shoulders; hands return to the sacrum along the sides of the body.

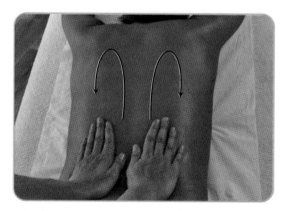

32 Alternate-hand effleurage: hands go up either side of the body out of sequence (this means you get a slight stretch to either side as you work).

33 Thousand-hand effleurage: first to one side, then to the other side of the body.

34 Reinforce hands (place one hand on top of the other); circular effleurage (of the buttock opposite the side you are standing).

35 Repeat alternate-hand effleurage, this time walking to the head of the couch as you work.

36 Thousand-hand effleurage down the body from the top of the couch, walking to the person's right side.

37 Reinforce hands; circular effleurage of the buttock opposite the side you are standing.

38 Standard effleurage of whole back; movements get lighter as you slow to finish.

39 Reflex strokes to finish.

casestudy: Massage for immune disorders

Chris was recovering from myalgic encephalomyelitis (ME), which he contracted following a series of cold viruses at a very stressful period in his life. Symptoms of ME include muscle pain, stiffness and overwhelming fatigue (coupled with insomnia) – a combination which brought Chris to massage to try to reduce the effects these symptoms were having on his health. As with other immune-related disorders, treating ME requires special consideration. First and foremost is that the treatment does not last as long as it would normally, as the person with ME will tend to tire more quickly. Second, it is advisable to stick to gentle effleurage movements and possibly a bit of kneading, but not to use any deeper or percussive strokes, as these can be both too stimulating and too intense for comfort.

Chris's first treatment only lasted 20 minutes and just involved effleurage of his legs, hands and arms. After 15 minutes he started to notice that he was feeling very tired and felt a mild headache coming on. We completed the treatment quickly, gave him a glass of water (which got rid of the headache) and agreed that he would decide when he was ready for the next treatment. After that first treatment, Chris noticed that he was able to sleep much more deeply and effectively for several days. He booked another treatment for five days after the first and we continued with the same pattern – that it would be primarily an effleurage treatment until he was able to manage an entire body treatment. In Chris's case, it was six weeks later (with an average of two treatments a week) before he could cope with an hour-long treatment, and another three weeks before any other strokes (apart from kneading) could be introduced without exhausting him. Twenty weeks into the treatment process, Chris was able to see that the benefits of the massage were now lasting a full week between treatments, which meant that we were able to reduce the frequency of the treatments (as well as adding more pressure to specific strokes). After 24 weeks, we reduced the treatments down to once a month or once every six weeks, which Chris now regards as a maintenance treatment or a health check, to make sure that he never gets that ill again.

Recovering from ME was a very long process for Chris and involved changes to his diet, lifestyle and working patterns, in addition to receiving regular massage. However, his recovery did bring about an increased awareness of how things (from food to exercise) affected him and he appeared to take great pleasure in the improvements that he noticed following the massage – that he was slowly able to take a longer treatment and to take more pressure, that he started sleeping more easily and feeling more alert for a couple of days after the treatment.

Massage during pregnancy

One of the most important aspects of massage during pregnancy is that you encourage the pregnant woman to get into a position for treatment where she is leaning forward or is almost on her hands and knees. Having her lie face down across a beanbag for the treatment is ideal, although sitting astride a chair is also fine. This particular position is very helpful at encouraging the baby to drop into the optimal delivery position, which, in turn, will help towards a shorter time in labour. If the pregnancy is advanced, ask the pregnant woman to lie on her side, get a pillow for her to rest her belly on and a second pillow to fold in half and place between her knees.

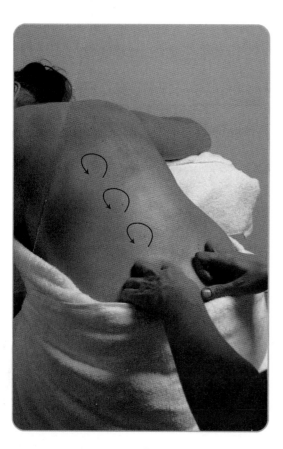

1 Effleurage from the sacrum up either side of the spine to the shoulders, circle over the shoulders and return down to the sacrum, moving gently along the sides of the body. Start with very light movements, getting progressively deeper.

2 Kneading along the sides of body and extensively over the top of the neck and shoulders.

3 Kneading to hands and arms, paying particular attention to hands if there is any swelling or oedema.

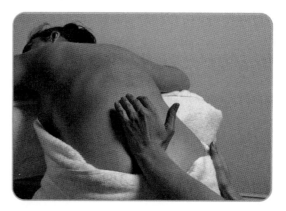

4 Heel-of-hand kneading into sacrum.

5 Knuckling into buttocks.

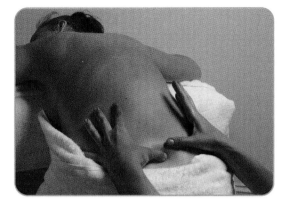

6 Finger frictions around the sacrum.

7 One-handed kneading to the neck and base of the skull.

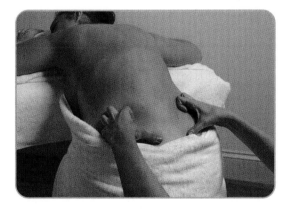

8 Petrissage up either side of the spine.

9 Petrissage around the shoulder blades.

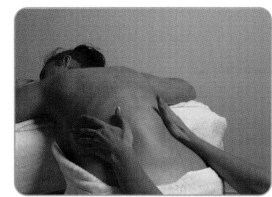

10 Lateralizing effleurage to lower back.

11 Effleurage to the whole of the upper leg.

12 Kneading to thigh and calf muscles.

13 Knuckling to thigh.

14 Frictions around ankle and knee.

15 Effleurage to foot.

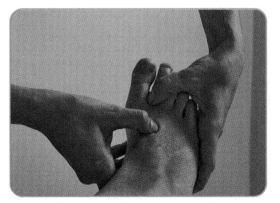

16 Frictions between toes.

73

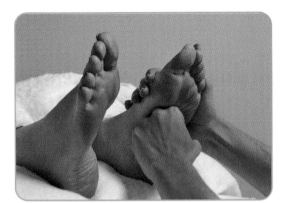

17 Knuckling to base of foot.

18 Heel-of-hand kneading to sacrum.

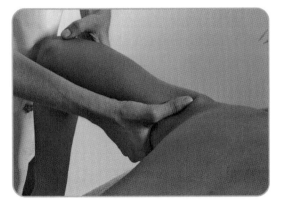

19 Additional frictions around shoulder blades.

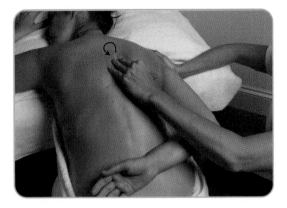

20 Mobilize and rotate shoulder.

21 Gentle circular effleurage to abdominal area (only after the first trimester and only if your friend feels comfortable receiving this treatment).

About perineal massage

The tissues of the perineum, found between the lower end of the vagina and the anus, will stretch and often tear (or need to be cut) during labour. Perineal massage is often suggested by midwives as a means of softening and preparing these tissues for labour. Regular treatment in the six weeks prior to delivery has been shown to minimize the necessity for an episiotomy, and reduces the chance of any tissue tearing during labour.

Massage during labour

Massage can be a great help to women in the earlier stages of labour, both to take their mind off the worsening contractions, as well as to help relieve pain, stress and discomfort.

- Effleurage from the sacrum up either side of the spine to the shoulders, circle over the shoulders and return to the sacrum, moving gently along the sides of the body. Start with very light movements, getting progressively deeper.
- Kneading over top of neck and shoulders – concentrate on this between contractions.
- Heel-of-hand kneading into sacrum – deepen pressure during any contractions.

- Knuckling into buttocks – again, deepen the pressure during contractions.
- One-handed kneading to the neck and the base of the skull.
- Repeat kneading and knuckling as often as desired.

Remember that as the labour deepens the mother will reach a point where she finds it unbearable to be touched. Do not take it personally when she makes it very clear that she wants you to stop treating her NOW. The important thing is that you carried out the treatment as and when it was needed and that it helped at the time.

Post-natal massage

The birth can be such a shock in some cases that the new mother may sometimes forget to pay as much attention to her physical and emotional needs after the baby is born as she did when she was preparing for the birth. Treatments shortly after the birth will vary according to the new mother's needs and what she experienced during the birth itself. A very invasive birth experience, such as a Caesarian section, will mean that she must avoid abdominal massage for a few months at least. However, other mothers will find that abdominal massage helps them to retrieve their pre-pregnancy muscle tone a little quicker. Back massages and facial treatments will benefit all new mothers, as will self-massage of the chest/breast area if they are having difficulties with breastfeeding, mastitis or weaning.

Self-massage of the chest area

This treatment method is very useful for those who experience painful or swollen breasts as a premenstrual symptom or during menstruation. It is also exceptionally useful when your breasts become engorged during breastfeeding or if you have a tendency to develop mastitis.

1 Apply a thin layer of oil to the chest area. If you are breastfeeding, it is important that this oil is fragrance-free and hypoallergenic (especially that it is not made from nut oils) – a good choice would be grapeseed oil. Make sure you avoid the nipple area when applying the oil.

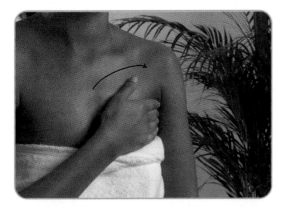

2 Effleurage around each breast, working up between the breasts (sternum to clavicle), then from sternum to armpit underneath the breasts, pausing each time you approach the armpit. There are key lymph nodes in the armpit which will help to remove any excess swelling following the massage.

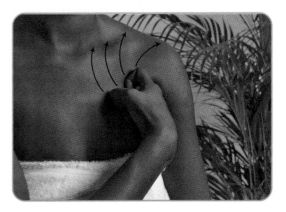

3 Gentle finger frictions around and over the breast tissue, working from the sternum over the top of the breast towards the armpit, then working the underside of the breast from sternum to armpit. If you find any nodules of tension or harder patches, this can be an indication of swollen or engorged mammary glands in breastfeeding women. Keep pressure gentle but firm, and work for slightly longer in this area until you start to feel the pain disperse. Do not be alarmed if you leak slightly during the treatment.

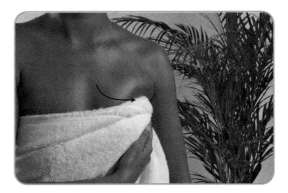

4 Swooping effleurage to finish, working from sternum to armpit, first above, then below each breast.

Baby massage

Baby massage is a specialist treatment in its own right; however, if you are confident in your massage treatment and want to try a short massage on your own infant, you can proceed with some additional cautions:

🐾 Pressure must be a lot lighter than normal. While you will be doing a little bit of kneading, most of the massage is effleurage and is designed to help you and your baby feel more comfortable.

🐾 Use a hypoallergenic carrier oil or one designed specifically for use with babies and toddlers.

🐾 Expect the massage to last for a short time. Most babies do not have the

patience of adults. Smaller infants will get hungry and need to nurse, usually after about 15–20 minutes. Most will fall asleep shortly after the treatment finishes.

🐾 Keep the room where you are working warm, as your baby will be naked during the treatment, and massage lowers body temperature.

🐾 You can expect a very young baby to empty his/her bladder or bowels during the treatment. Keep cleaning materials to hand.

🐾 Older babies will wriggle and move off once they are bored. Let them decide how long the treatment will be.

1 Start with baby face up. Make lots of eye contact, smile and ensure your hands are warm before you begin to apply oil.

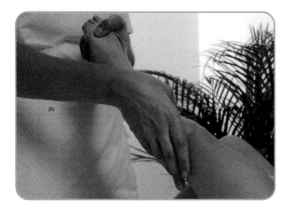

2 Apply oil to both legs, using swooping effleurage movements.

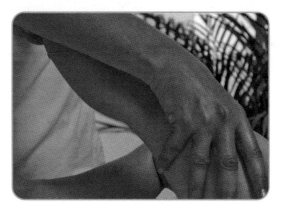

3 Progress slowly into kneading, first of one leg, then the other, then both legs at the same time. Concentrate most of the kneading in the thigh area.

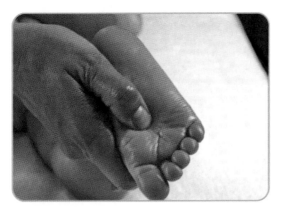

4 Petrissage to the base of the feet.

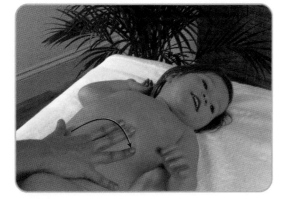

5 Gentle circular effleurage in a clockwise motion to the abdomen, using one hand only.

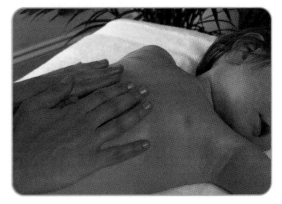

6 Using both hands, effleurage up the sternum, over the shoulders and down the arms. Repeat several times.

7 Gradually alter your effleurage, letting it become firmer until it develops into kneading.

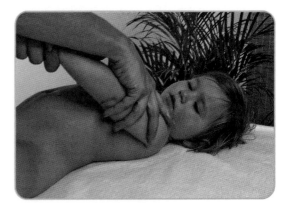

8 Kneading to each arm in turn.

effleurage massage

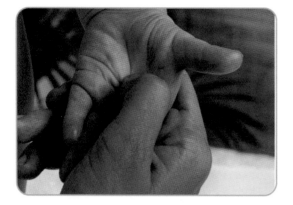

9 Petrissage to the palms.

10 Roll the baby over and apply oil to the back and buttocks.

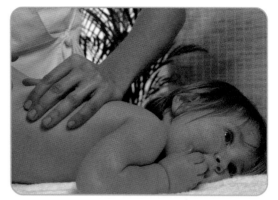

12 Kneading to back and buttocks.

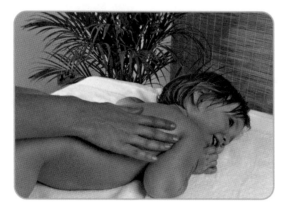

11 Effleurage to whole back and buttocks.

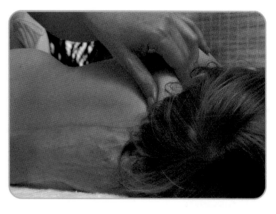

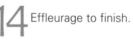

13 Kneading with fingertips to shoulder area and then to hip area.

14 Effleurage to finish.

FAQs: About effleurage massage

Surely the more pressure you put into a massage movement, the better it is? Why should effleurage remain light?

Effleurage acts as an assessing stroke, helping you to discover areas of muscle tension and helping the client to become accustomed to your touch. People have different preferences where pressure is concerned. These preferences are also subject to change: if they are feeling fragile one day, they will want a nurturing rather than an invigorating session. Most of the people you will treat may need to build up to the most appropriate pressure. Appropriate pressure for effleurage is when you can see the skin (and underlying muscle) move or ripple ahead of your hands as you are working.

Why do I have to be so gentle with my friend who has ME? He actually needs the energy boost of a stimulating treatment, not a relaxing one.

Both ME and post-viral fatigue are misleading in this respect. Yes, the person with these conditions wants to feel energized (or just to have some energy again, as in some cases they have forgotten what it feels like not to be tired all the time); however, their body is still recovering from a very exhausting and debilitating condition. Massage for them may be the most exercise that their body has experienced in some time. Regular treatment can help them to get fit enough to have the energizing and stimulating treatment you want to offer them. However, you should start slowly and build up gradually. Keep treatments gentle and short and check with your friend how he feels in the few days after treatment to give you an idea of how he is responding. You can expect that after the first few treatments he will feel exhausted the next day, or possibly for several days afterwards. Do not provide a stimulating or vigorous treatment until he is able to take a full body effleurage treatment (lasting around one hour) and feel physically well for at least a couple of days after treatment. It is also positively beneficial not to provide a stimulating treatment at all – a gentle treatment will work just as effectively for someone who has ME as a stimulating one would for another person.

effleurage massage

How can I adapt my baby massage to cope with constipation? What about colic?
While it is unusual for small babies to experience constipation, when they have it, you will hear about it! Try raising the knees and legs into a vertical position and holding them with one hand. Using your other hand, place it over the lower abdomen and press gently, while rocking the knees to one side, then the other. This gives a gentle wringing effect to the colon, which can help to move faecal matter. If you do this, make sure you do not do it immediately after a meal, as the infant will bring up what they ate if their stomach is full. For colic, one of the most effective massage methods is to hold the baby face down over your forearm, so that the heel of your hand presses into their lower abdomen. Use the palm of your other hand to knead the back, particularly the lower back. This pressure is often very comforting to a colicky child and will sometimes assist in winding.

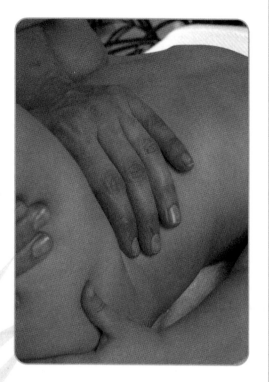

massage in practice

The more you practise your massage movements, the easier and more effective they will become. Eventually, you will find that the movements flow into each other and that you are able to maintain the rhythm and pressure desirable, regardless of any distractions. You will also find that it becomes easier to identify which movements are going to be most effective for the person receiving the massage, and you will have the confidence to develop a treatment tailored to suit individual needs.

8 chapter

legs and feet

The legs and feet are the ideal place to start working when you want to practise your percussion strokes – as long as you have checked that there are no contraindications to treatment. The majority of people benefit from more invigorating massage strokes in this area as this will warm up the muscles prior to exercise and can reduce any pain following exercise or as a result of standing for long periods. This is also an area that people can sometimes be very self-conscious about if they feel their legs are not as toned as they would like them to be. You must be particularly careful to check for any contraindications on the legs and feet, however – bruises, surface veins, varicose veins and any potential injuries in the area must be considered before commencing treatment.

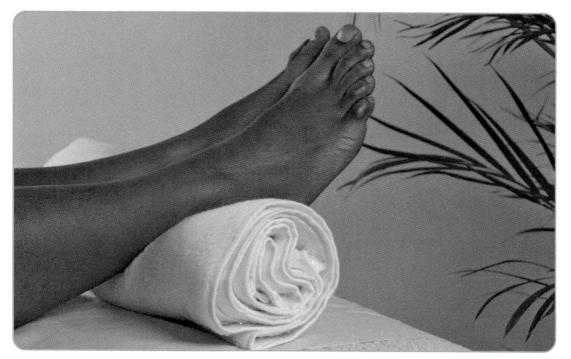

Leg massage

Supine

1 Expose the leg and apply carrier oil in smooth strokes over the entire surface of the leg.

2 Effleurage three strokes each of hands opposing and hand leading hand.

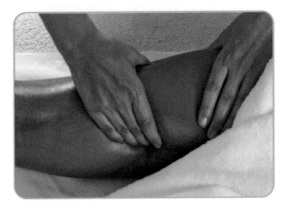

3 Kneading to whole of thigh area, working from inner thigh to outer thigh.

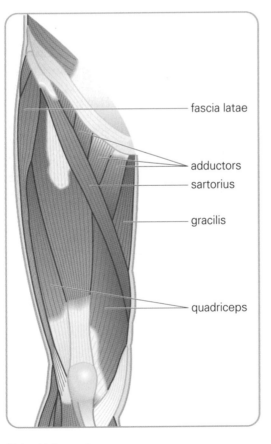

- fascia latae
- adductors
- sartorius
- gracilis
- quadriceps

Major thigh muscles

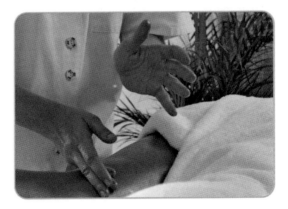

4 Hacking to thigh area – be careful to avoid knee.

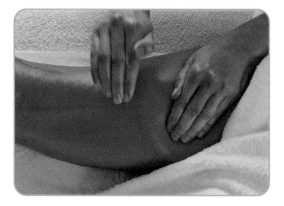

5 Cupping to thigh area.

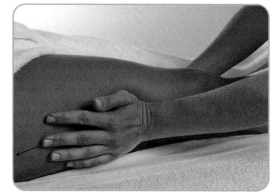

7 Deep heel-of-hand drainage to iliotibial band – start from the belly of the quadriceps muscle, especially if the person has very sensitive knees or does not have a great deal of muscle development in this area.

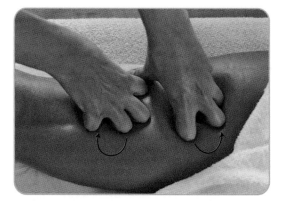

6 Knuckling to thigh area.

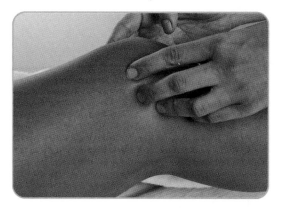

8 Finger frictions around the knee – work around the knee and then into the popliteal region (back of the knee).

massage in essence

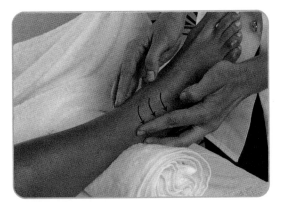

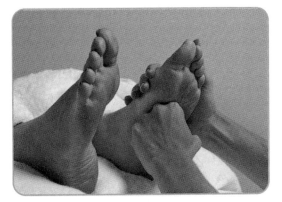

9 Gentle effleurage to ankles; finger frictions around the ankle.

10 Effleurage to the foot.

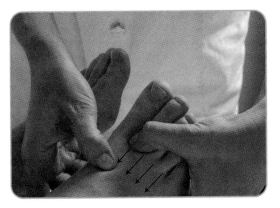

11 Finger frictions between the metatarsals.

12 Deep pressure to base of the foot, first with your fingers, in five strips down from toes to heel, then using your fist into instep.

13 Repeat effleurage, gradually becoming lighter to finish.

14 Repeat for other leg.

Prone

15 Expose the leg and apply carrier oil.

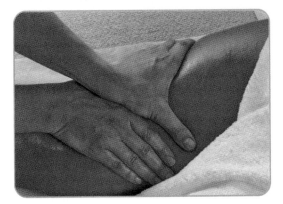

16 Effleurage three strokes each of hands opposing and hand leading hand.

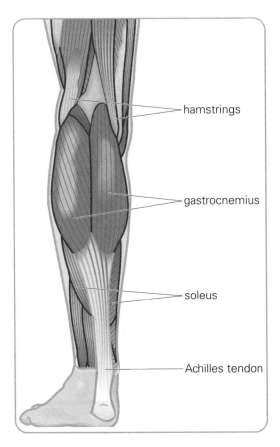

The main posterior leg muscles

17 Kneading to whole of thigh area, working from inner thigh to outer thigh.

18 Kneading to calf area.

19 Hacking to thigh area – you can repeat this for the calf area if you feel confident and you know that your hacking is very light, also making sure that the person you are treating does not have any vascular conditions such as deep-vein thrombosis, severe bruising or varicose veins.

20 Cupping to thigh area.

21 Knuckling to thigh area.

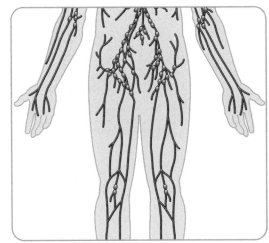

Lymphatic vessels and nodes on the thigh

22 Lymphatic drainage to thigh area – divide thigh into three areas and work with your thumb in deep strokes along the medial, then intermediate, then lateral portions of the hamstrings. When you do this right (and assuming the person has some cellulite), it will feel as if you are popping bubble wrap when you work.

23 Deep heel-of-hand drainage to side of leg.

24 Additional kneading to gastrocnemius and soleus.

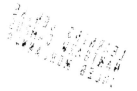

massage in essence

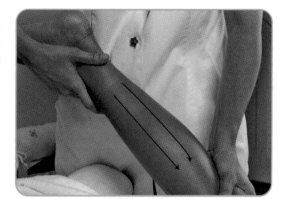

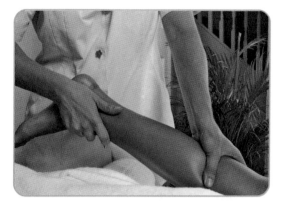

25 Lymph drainage to gastrocnemius and soleus – raise the lower leg to allow gravity to assist you. Work in three strips, from medial to intermediate, then lateral portions of the gastrocnemius. When you work the intermediate portion of the muscle, it will feel as if the two heads of the gastrocnemius separate for your thumb to work through.

26 Raise knee to vertical position, draining with the whole of the palm into the popliteal region, then using your knuckles to drain the thigh area.

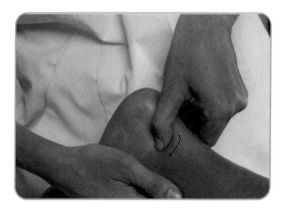

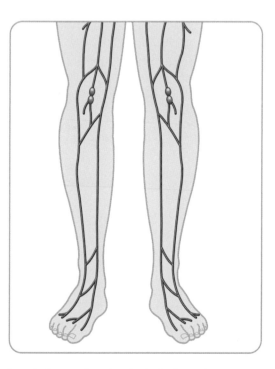

Lymphatic vessels and nodes in the lower leg

27 Lower leg somewhat, then use fingers and thumbs to provide frictions to the heel and the attachment points for the Achilles tendon.

28 Repeat effleurage, gradually becoming lighter to finish.

29 Repeat for other leg.

casestudy: Oedema as a result of circulation disorders

Mabel was 75 when she first came for massage. She had severe oedema around her ankles and lower legs as a result of a heart condition. Although she was taking tablets, which did reduce the water retention, her son had suggested she try massage to see if it could assist further.

In Mabel's case, all percussion movements were contraindicated. Apart from the swelling in her lower legs, she was very frail, had dry, papery skin and was quickly exhausted. Treating Mabel involved using a rich carrier oil and primarily slow, smooth effleurage strokes, some gentle kneading and very gentle finger and thumb frictions around the affected areas. At first, Mabel found the frictions quite painful, even when they were kept light. This appeared to be because she was retaining so much fluid in these areas that her skin felt tight – almost to bursting point. When she found an area painful, we would return to effleurage before trying again. After three sessions (within two weeks) she noticed a distinct improvement – there was much less swelling and Mabel felt significantly less tired at the end of the treatment and for a day or so afterwards. I encouraged her to start doing a little light exercise, as this would also help to reduce the swelling (muscles contracting in and around the area that was swollen would help to move the oedema back towards the heart). Mabel found walking her dog for 20 minutes a day was the most she could comfortably do, although she reported that she felt far more positive and refreshed as a result of getting back into doing this, where for some time she had been relying on others to walk her dog for her. Once she had started to engage in a little more exercise, Mabel found that it did help to reduce the oedema to the extent that she could reduce the number of massage treatments she had down to a half-hour treatment once every three weeks. This treatment would only concentrate on her legs.

Treating cellulite

Some professional therapists and medical practitioners will argue that cellulite does not really exist, or that what the health and beauty industries describe as cellulite – a distinctive orange-peel effect on the skin – is not cellulite at all. Whatever your opinion on the subject, we can agree on the following:

- when we have skin and muscle tissue that appears dimpled in this way, we do not always like its appearance;

- we can never completely destroy fat cells (just empty them and make them pack flatter until they are given the substances required to make them expand again);

- exercise which concentrates on toning muscles in problem areas will improve the appearance of the skin and muscle in these areas – massage is one of these exercises which is particularly effective;

- things which improve blood flow to these problem areas (including skin brushing and vigorous massage) will also improve the body's ability to remove toxins which are collecting in these areas;
- changes to diet and lifestyle can also help to improve the appearance of skin and muscle in any area, but are particularly effective when treating cellulite.

Treating cellulite with massage is a very popular treatment, particularly after Christmas, when people want to detox and start thinking about getting into bathing suits in the very near future. The treatment is so vigorous that the massage therapist will also get a proper workout. An additional advantage is that this treatment is very easy to adapt to working on yourself – if you accompany it with appropriate changes to diet and lifestyle, you can see visible results within a matter of weeks.

Cellulite massage

Use the massage routine outlined for the legs above as a guide, but make the following changes:

- Dry skin brushing before the treatment to increase the circulation to the skin immediately.
- If you are using a pre-blended massage oil which contains essential oils, pick one

which is labelled as being for either detox or muscular aches and pains. Both of these will contain essential oils that are particularly effective at stimulating the circulation to the legs, which will also improve the effects of your treatment. Remember that with any use of essential oils you must read the instructions on the bottle and avoid any contraindications that are highlighted. (For example, a lot of the essential oils used for detox or muscular aches and pains are not advisable if you are pregnant, breastfeeding, under the age of 12 or have sensitive or damaged skin. Various medications can also be affected by these treatments.)

- Keep all movements, even the effleurage, fast and vigorous.
- Lengthen the time you spend on hacking and cupping. With practice, you should be able to keep this up for at least five minutes on each leg (that's five minutes of hacking, followed by five minutes of cupping).
- If you are treating yourself for cellulite, do the treatment at least twice a day.
- Do *not* do this treatment at all if you have varicose veins, any form of thrombosis or blood-clotting disorder, severe bruising or similar cardiovascular conditions.

Self-massage for cellulite

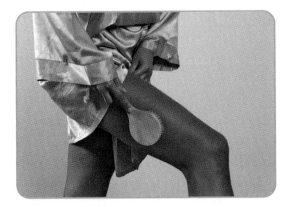

1 Skin brushing over dry skin – keep this vigorous (but not painful) and make sure the strokes go towards the heart.

2 Apply oil to the entire leg and as much of the buttock as you can comfortably reach while sitting down, with ankle crossed over knee.

3 Vigorous effleurage over the lower leg, followed by as much as you can reach of the upper leg.

4 Frictions around ankle.

5 Kneading to lower leg.

6 Cupping to lower leg (medial side of gastrocnemius and soleus).

7 Repeat kneading, taking strokes into the popliteal node.

8 Palmar drainage to lower leg – this is most easily done if you raise the leg.

9 Kneading to thigh area – as much as you can reach.

10 Knuckling to thigh area.

11 Hacking to thigh area (medial side) – try to maintain this for at least five minutes.

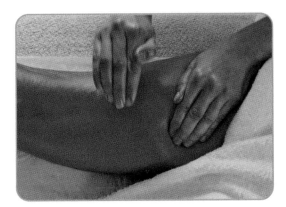

12 Cupping to thigh area (medial side), then stand to do cupping to lateral side and to the buttock area) – maintain this for at least five minutes. If it feels uncomfortable, return to effleurage and kneading for a while, then repeat cupping.

13 Palmar drainage towards inguinal nodes.

14 Repeat effleurage over whole leg.

15 Repeat routine for other leg.

Treating sciatica

Sciatica is the term used to refer to neuralgia, or nerve pain, of the sciatic nerve. While it can develop for a number of reasons, it is always very painful and occasionally will prevent the person from sitting, lying or walking comfortably. Bouts of sciatica will come and

93

go, and the person suffering with it will often be able to link the sciatica to activities they have carried out or, in some cases, to stress. What usually happens in sciatica is that the deep muscles underlying the gluteals go into spasm and contract down on the nerve, causing pain and tingling, which can travel down the leg. Sometimes this is made worse by swelling or inflammation around the sacrum or additional muscles going into spasm in the buttock and elsewhere on the leg, particularly at the back of the leg.

Sciatica will respond well to massage, but you do need to take additional care in the treatment process and get plenty of feedback from the person you are treating. (Make sure that you never go beyond a 'good hurt' – where the pressure you are applying feels like it is doing some good; if it hurts too much, you must stop what you are doing.) Furthermore, you have to spend longer working around the top of the hip, sacrum and the sides of the buttock to really ease the pain. I have found the following treatment to be very effective.

1 Passive stretches to gluteal muscles and the lumbar region. Reinforce your hands (one hand over the other) and place them to one side of the sacrum; lean onto your hands and let the muscle hold your weight for up to one minute. Move to repeat stretch to the buttock opposite the side you are standing.

2 Expose gluteus medius down to the gluteal fold, standing to one side of the client – all the movements you are about to do will be done to the buttock opposite the side you are standing. Apply oil.

3 Start with kneading – keep your movements rhythmic and slow, gradually picking up some speed and adding a bit more pressure as you feel the muscles warm up and relax beneath your hands.

4 Stretching to piriformis – using one hand to lift the bulk of the gluteal muscle (this forces it to relax); work with side of thumb and heel of other hand to push deep into the muscle, moving from the sacrum to the head of the femur.

5 Knuckling to gluteus medius, working in small circular movements from sacrum to head of femur and along (and slightly below) the iliac crest (curved portion of the upper hip bone).

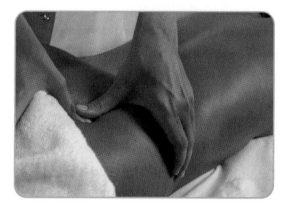

6 Petrissage in lines across the gluteus medius, working in straight lines initially (from the sacrum to the side of the hip and the origin of the tensor fascia lata, following the line of the iliac crest and finishing at the border marked by the towel covering the client).

7 Repeat kneading and knuckling to whole of gluteal region.

8 Petrissage on a diagonal, working from the sacrum to the head of the femur, along the line of the piriformis.

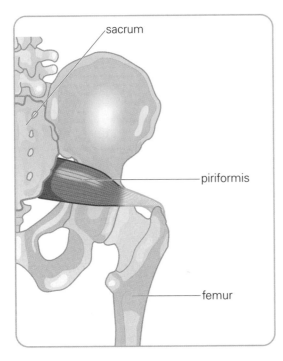

Location of piriformis in relation to sacrum and femur

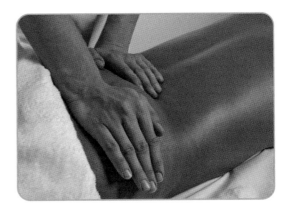

9 Deep heel-of-hand stretching to gluteals – reinforce hands if appropriate.

10 Light hacking to gluteals (assuming that the person is *not* having a flare-up of their sciatica when you are treating them – leave this move out if they are currently in pain).

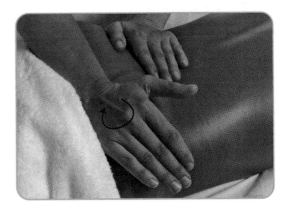

11 Heel-of-hand rotations to piriformis and head of femur.

12 Petrissage to sacroiliac joint and to whole of sacrum.

13 Kneading to finish.

14 Repeat for other buttock.

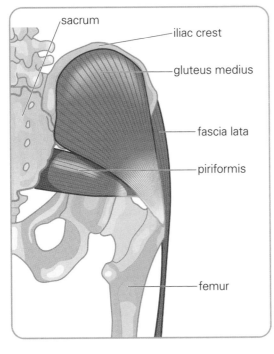

The gluteal region

95

FAQs: About leg massage

When I do my hacking and cupping to the thighs, the towels always roll down my friend's legs. How do I manage the towels so that they stay in place and I do not have to keep adjusting them?

You need to roll the towels tighter when you expose the leg. Try rolling the longitudinal towel in on itself in a tight roll, and folding the transverse towel back as well as tucking it slightly under your friend's body.

How can I do an effective treatment for sciatica on my mother when she wears big knickers?

You have two choices. First, you can do the top part of the massage by lowering her knickers to the gluteal fold while she is covered by the towel. You can try to tuck the towel into the leg of the knickers and raise them when doing the lower part of the leg massage. The second choice is to raise the subject with her, suggesting that she either wears skimpy underwear when she has a treatment or foregoes the underwear altogether. If you raise the subject after you have tried doing the massage over her usual lingerie, she will be aware of any problems you had and may be prepared to make it easier for you in the future.

How would I know if someone has deep-vein thrombosis? I understand that it is a contraindication to massage in the legs.

Deep-vein thrombosis (DVT) is a blood clot that is found in the big veins deep within the muscles of the leg, usually appearing initially in the calf muscles. The thrombosis becomes dangerous when the blood clot breaks away from where it formed and starts to travel up the legs towards the heart, lungs and brain. If it is not caught early enough and dealt with appropriately, it can be exceedingly dangerous.

The short answer to this question is that you will not always know, so if you are at all worried or something you see or feel

Additional variation

When you are doing the rest of the leg massage in the prone position, expose the leg high on the buttocks and add in the following strokes:

- Additional hand-leading-hand effleurage, leaning into the stroke so that you push your hands against the outer curve of the gluteus maximus to stretch this area.
- Kneading to the outer curve of the gluteus maximus.
- Pounding to the gluteals.
- Knuckling to the outer curve of the gluteus maximus, encouraging additional stretching to this area.
- Heel-of-hand rotations to the outer curve of the gluteus maximus.

does not seem normal, you should not proceed with the massage. However, key things to look out for which *sometimes* indicate the possibility of a DVT include:

- variation in skin temperature between one calf and the other (one seems hot and the other cold, or parts of the same leg seem hot and cold);

- pain on walking (and the pain is not constant);

- swelling in feet, ankles or knees, especially if it is only on one side;

- swelling in the calf muscles themselves, especially only on one side;

- a recent spell of sitting or lying very still for a long period of time (including hospitalization and/or airline travel).

What do massage therapists mean when they talk about how massage helps to eliminate toxins from the body?

The short definition for toxin is a poisonous substance. This could include bacteria, pollutants (such as carbon monoxide from car exhaust, lead, coal dust, arsenic, mercury or other heavy metals), as well as the by-products of the break down of food, any medications or supplements being taken and the waste products produced by the body as a result of cell metabolism.

Massage helps eliminate toxins by reducing the symptoms which indicate that toxins are present (usually things like headaches, fatigue, lethargy, pain, lymphatic congestion, oedema or swelling). Also, by improving the circulation, it helps to get additional oxygen to the body cells, stimulate the key organs involved in detoxification (the liver and kidneys), reduce oedema and improve the elimination of waste via the bowels, lungs and bladder.

hands and arms

The hands and arms are often neglected as part of a massage treatment, usually because people would like you to concentrate on their back or legs (if these need toning). However, treatment here can be profoundly effective, especially in cases involving repetitive strain, tennis elbow or frozen shoulder. Work in this area is also very effective at improving muscle tone in the upper arms and should be an essential part of any self-help routine by the therapist, as these are the areas that will take the brunt of your work, especially if you are not watching your posture and using your body effectively. Most of the routine suggested for the arms can be adapted for self-use; try treating yourself once a week, or more often if you know you are prone to feeling pain or have poor circulation in your hands.

Arms

1 Expose arm, hold arm by the wrist and lean back to apply gentle stretch to shoulder joint.

2 Apply oil over entire arm and shoulder.

3 Effleurage over entire arm.

4 Kneading to forearm.

massage in essence

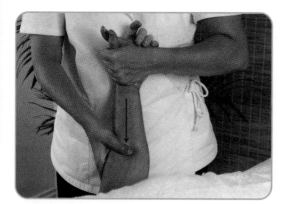

5 Drainage to forearm.

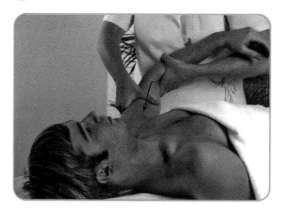

6 One-handed kneading to upper arm – raise arm and work from the top of the couch.

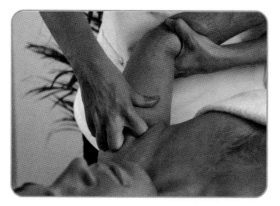

7 Knuckling to upper arm, especially to deltoids and attachment points for pectorals.

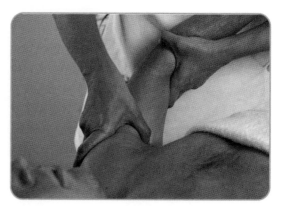

8 Drainage to upper arm.

9 Double-handed drainage around the shoulder.

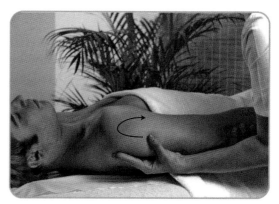

10 Passive rotation to the shoulder – grasp the upper arm in one hand and the elbow with the other, lifting and rotating the shoulder in a shrugging movement.

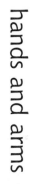

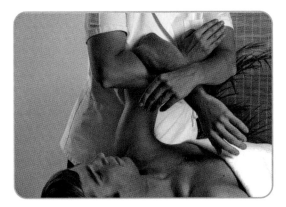

12 Vertical effleurage of the hand.

13 Horizontal effleurage of the hand.

14 Finger frictions between metacarpals.

15 Petrissage to palmar surface, especially in the region of the carpals.

16 Petrissage to each finger, plus gentle stretching to joints.

17 Reflex strokes to finish.

11 Passive stretch to the shoulder – raise the arm, folding the forearm over your arm, and by standing on your toes you will lift the arm away from the massage couch, allowing for a passive stretch to the rhomboids and rotator cuff muscles and relaxing the pectoral muscles at the same time.

casestudy: Repetitive strain injury (RSI)

After 20 years working as a bricklayer, and two fractures (both to the same wrist), Alan has developed a serious repetitive strain injury in his right forearm and wrist. The severity of the condition depends on the amount and type of work he is doing, and is made worse by those occasions when he is required to pull down walls or break up bricks. Alan first tried massage as a means of pain relief for his RSI when a friend asked him to be a case study for the massage course she was doing. While he reports that the regular massages (which included extra attention to his arms and hands) did help, the work in between sessions, when he massaged his own arm for up to 20 minutes a day, was more effective. This treatment, which he did every day for two months, is a variation on the hand and arm routine below.

1 Effleurage to the whole arm and shoulder, making sure that you warm up the muscles and skin effectively.

2 One-handed kneading to the palm, wrist, forearm, upper arm and shoulder. Keep the kneading rhythmic and almost wring the muscles laterally when you are working.

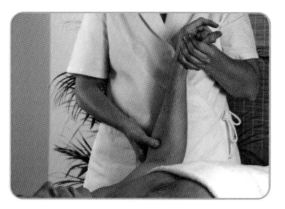

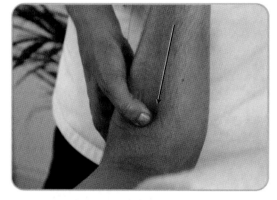

3 'Hooking' with your thumb along the extensor muscles, each in turn, working from the carpals in the wrist, up to and including the elbow. (Hooking is a term used in reflexology to describe a caterpillar-like movement with your thumb along the length of the muscle.) Keep these movements as deep as you can comfortably manage.

4 Petrissage (rotations this time) along the same muscles in turn, working from carpals to elbow.

5 Repeat petrissage, but this time, as you are working, tilt your wrist with each movement, which will mean that your petrissage goes deeper – this can be quite painful initially. If you are trying this for the first time, you may want to leave this movement out until you have seen some improvement.

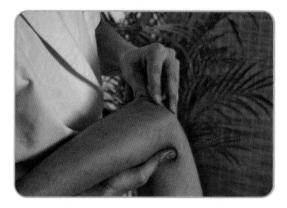

6 Petrissage into the oleocranon process (the gap at the base of the humerus where it forms a joint with the radius and ulna). This can be quite painful if there is a lot of swelling around the elbow or if you have a history of bursitis (inflammation of the bursae – in the elbow this is sometimes called tennis elbow).

7 Petrissage up the lateral side of the upper arm (along the triceps and deltoids) and into the lateral side of the acromion process – most of the muscles that help to rotate the shoulder are attached around here, so the more petrissage you do, the more movement you will achieve later.

8 Knuckling to the anterior deltoid, coracobrachialis and the insertion points of the pectoralis major.

9 Petrissage to the upper parts of the trapezius and sternocleidomastoid, moving towards the neck and paying particular attention to trigger points – areas of painful or stiff muscle that are surrounded by softer tissue.

10 Kneading followed by effleurage to finish.

FAQs: About hand and arm massage

How do I protect myself from injury when doing massage? I have done three treatments in the last two days and my hands hurt.

To get effectively fit for massage and stay that way, you need to build up the strength in your hands and arms by massaging your own hands daily, and start to be a bit more aware of when they are hurting (and stopping work before they hurt too much) and adapt any movements that are particularly likely to hurt your hands. Try adjusting how you move your hands, keeping wrists straight rather than at angles when you work. If your thumbs are really sore (usually with petrissage), try either reinforcing them when you work (one thumb over the other to add pressure without pain), or switch to knuckling as far as possible. You can also do additional work with your forearms or elbows to take the place of working extensively with your thumbs.

Can massage do anything to improve my nails?

Yes, it can, particularly if you are massaging other people regularly as well as massaging your own hands and nails. The vegetable oil you use to carry out a treatment will provide some of the essential nutrients that your nails need to become healthier (and most of the carrier oils are mildly antiseptic and anti-fungal, so if you have a tendency towards nail-bed infections, these can improve with regular use of oil). Furthermore, if you are doing your massage properly, you will be paring your nails regularly and keeping them very short. This will help to improve their health.

My son has a frozen shoulder. Can I do anything to help him using massage?

Frozen shoulder is a term that is sometimes used to refer to injuries, damage or strain to the rotator cuff muscles. These muscles (the supraspinatus, infraspinatus, teres major, teres minor and subscapularis) lie over and around the scapula and are involved in rotating the shoulder (along with the deltoid). Your son probably finds some movements of the shoulder either difficult or painful, and he may have difficulty lifting his arm in certain directions. The most useful movements to help ease the pain and discomfort of rotator cuff injuries are those which bring blood to the surface around the shoulder joint and which work into the muscles which are tense. Double-handed effleurage around the shoulder joint (looks like you are sawing away at the joint) is a great help, as is knuckling over the pectoral muscles, and petrissage around and over the tendons for the rotator cuff muscles.

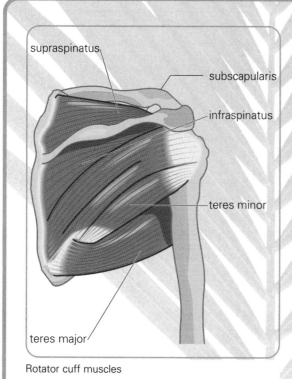

supraspinatus

subscapularis

infraspinatus

teres minor

teres major

Rotator cuff muscles

You can feel these tendons near the lateral edge of the scapula, around the point at which it is attached to the acromion process.

I have flabby upper arms. Will massage help to tone them up?

Massage will help tone up any muscles that are treated. However, the most effective way in which massage can tone upper arms is if you are giving the massages, rather than receiving them. If this is something you would like to benefit from while carrying out massage treatments, make sure that your massage table (if you are using one) is slightly lower than usual, keep your elbows locked while you are doing any effleurage, knuckling or petrissage (this means that your triceps brachii will be contracted for these movements) and ensure you do plenty of regular hacking and cupping.

back, neck and shoulders

Most of the people you practise on will be more than happy if you want to spend more time working over the back. It is worth really practising this treatment until you feel very satisfied with the response you get. Keep the pressure firm and the movements rhythmic to get the best effects.

Neck and shoulders (in supine position)

1 Effleurage over upper pectoral muscles, upper trapezius, deltoids and the back of the neck.

2 Back-and-forth effleurage of trapezius.

3 Thousand-hand effleurage to one side of the neck, then the other.

4 Knuckling to top of pectorals, deltoids and trapezius (do not go below the third rib, as this can be very painful, especially if the person you are massaging has large or painful breasts).

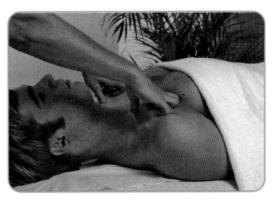

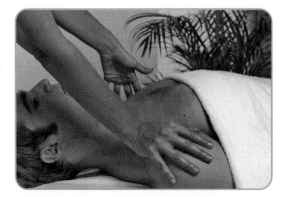

5 Stretching out to pectoral muscles (place your hands on each shoulder and lean first on one shoulder, then on the next, in a see-saw motion).

6 Petrissage to trapezius and supraspinatus, working into any trigger points (see page 111) that you find. Movements should be in small circles, then in straight lines, starting from the root of the neck and moving outwards towards the acromion process.

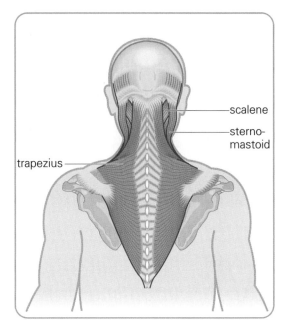

Cervical muscles

7 Petrissage to cervical muscles, moving from the root of the neck to the occipital.

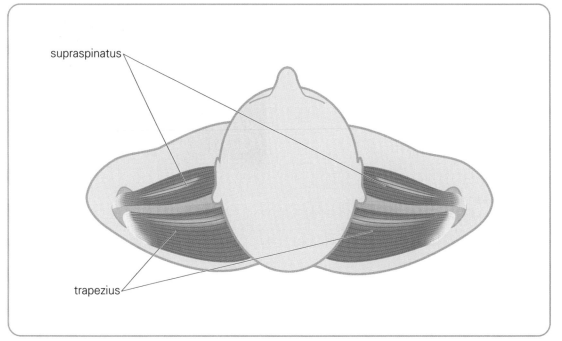

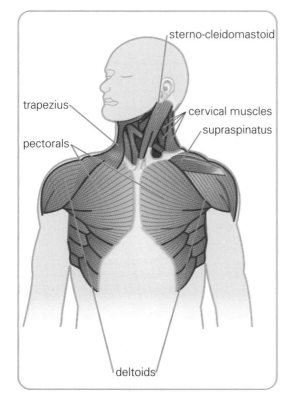

sterno-cleidomastoid

trapezius

cervical muscles

supraspinatus

pectorals

deltoids

Muscles in neck and shoulder region

8 Repeat effleurage to both sides of the back of the neck, stretching the muscles slightly by gently leaning back each time your hands come to the occipital.

Back and buttocks

9 Standing to the person's left, expose the back and upper buttocks and apply oil.

10 Standard effleurage up the back, along the erector spinae muscles, from the sacrum to the top of the shoulders, returning along the sides of the body.

11 Fountain effleurage.

12 Kneading to the opposite side of the body to where you are standing, from hips to shoulder.

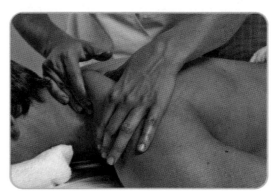

13 Kneading across shoulders, first right shoulder, then both shoulders, then left shoulder.

14 Kneading of left side of the body, from shoulder to hip.

15 Repeat effleurage.

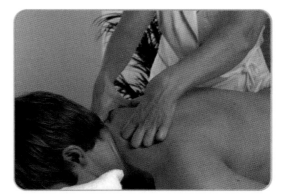

16 Knuckling over entire back, concentrating on areas of tension, particularly around the trapezius, levator scapulae and rhomboids.

17 Petrissage over erector spinae and any other areas of tension.

massage in essence

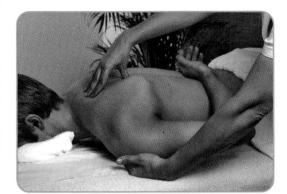

18 Working with the arm closest to you, place the client's wrist into the small of their back, getting them to drop their elbow so that the medial edge of the scapula rises, exposing the rhomboids. Petrissage to the rhomboids and supraspinatus.

19 Repeat effleurage and kneading.

20 Reinforce hands – circular effleurage to buttock opposite the side you are standing.

21 Kneading to buttock opposite the side you are standing.

22 Heel-of-hand stretching to piriformis.

23 Petrissage in straight lines across gluteus medius.

24 Repeat kneading to buttocks.

25 Repeat kneading to side of the body.

26 Alternate-hand effleurage to back, walking up to the top of the couch.

27 Petrissage to upper trapezius from top of the couch.

28 Thousand-hand effleurage – first to one side, then to the other side of the body.

29 Walk to the other side of the body and repeat steps 4–18.

30 Repeat petrissage to erector spinae.

31 Vibrations to erector spinae.

32 Standard effleurage of whole back – movements get lighter as you slow to finish.

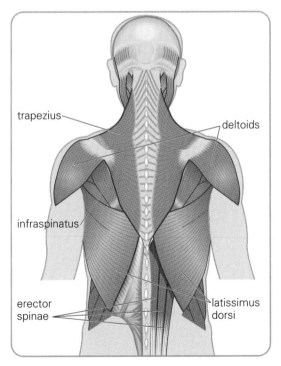

The major muscles of the back

33 Reflex strokes to finish.

casestudy: Muscle tension headaches

Ian regularly gets tension headaches, although they recently started getting worse, with occasional migraine-style symptoms which occurred mostly at the weekends. A couple of years ago he used to get massages once a week in order to keep himself in good physical condition. He stopped getting the treatments when he changed jobs, as his new job involved a great deal of travel and less regular hours. While Ian had noticed that the headaches were getting worse and were linked to problems at work, he did not consider massage until he found he was completely debilitated by blinding headaches once a week, almost always on a Friday evening or a Saturday. Treating Ian effectively involved making an agreement with him that he would have treatments once a week for four weeks, but that he would also massage his own shoulders and neck every day for ten minutes – five in the morning and five in the evening. He was also told not to expect the headaches to disappear immediately, but that it would take perseverance on his part for at least a month.

There is a point at which muscle tension headaches can cause migraine-like symptoms. In Ian's case, what was happening was that as tension built up in the week, his muscles would get tighter, making him feel very uncomfortable. As the muscles contracted, they were pressing down on the associated nerves (causing pain) and blood vessels (constricting the blood flow to the area). At the end of the week, as Ian relaxed and looked forward to a weekend off, so the muscles would relax and the blood, constricted for so long, would flow into the muscles around the head, resulting in the characteristic pounding sensation.

Ian's first treatment took place on a Saturday, when the tension headache was very bad. Having discussed how his lifestyle contributed to his headaches, we agreed that he would start massaging his own shoulders and neck daily from that day onwards, and that he would come for his next treatment on a Wednesday, in the hope that we would be able to reduce the tension to the extent that it did not build up to extreme levels by the weekend. The treatment mainly involved kneading, knuckling and thumb petrissage to the upper trapezius and cervical muscles, as well as some stretching to the neck and shoulders. The treatment also included finger frictions to the scalp in order to ease any underlying tension in the occipitofrontalis muscles (which are where most muscle tension headaches arise), as well as some gentle petrissage to the sides of the face and jaw.

back, neck and shoulders

massage in essence

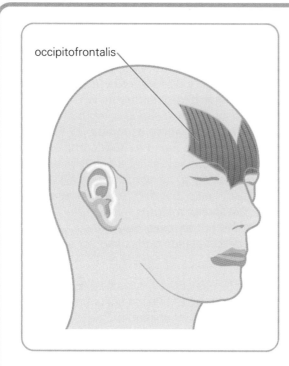

occipitofrontalis

Occipitofrontalis muscle

At Ian's second treatment, he reported that while the headache was not as intense, he still felt rough until Monday, when he returned to work. However, he had kept up with his short self-massages and there was a noticeable improvement in the muscle tone in the areas he had been working, which were much more pliable. We continued with the same form of treatment for two more weeks before Ian was able to confirm that he had no more migraine-style symptoms and that his tension headaches were also getting less frequent. He found the self-help massage so useful that he had started to increase the length of time that he did the massage for and was also able to treat himself in his lunch break occasionally. Having realized how his job was affecting him physically, he began to consider seriously whether he wanted to stay in it. This resulted in him deciding that while he loved his work, he needed to travel less and concentrate on making sure that he built relaxing activities back into his life.

FAQs: About back, neck and shoulder massage

What is a trigger point? How do I get rid of them? Do I want to get rid of them?

'Trigger point' is a term body therapists (massage therapists and many other practitioners who work on the physical body, including osteopaths and chiropractors) tend to use to describe a tight, contracted nodule of muscle which is surrounded by softer tissue. This develops as a result of the body's exposure to one or more stressors, which might include injury, toxins, heavy or repetitive physical activity or emotional stress. The body responds to these stressors by sending messages via the nervous system to the muscles and blood vessels in or around the affected region. This will cause muscle spasms and often constrict the blood vessels. If these are not treated often enough, physical changes can occur to the muscle which will then develop these trigger points. The most common areas for trigger points to develop are in the levator scapulae, supraspinatus and rhomboid muscles. You can reduce the size of a trigger point (and the pain associated with it) through massage (mainly petrissage and stretching movements), but this is usually temporary unless you deal with whatever stressors caused the trigger point to develop in the first place.

My partner has kyphosis. How can I help to improve her posture and make it comfortable for her to receive treatment?

Kyphosis is an exaggerated curvature of the thoracic spine. It can occur for a number of reasons – poor posture (perhaps years spent slumped over a computer, a desk, a sewing machine or something similar), osteoporosis in later life or,

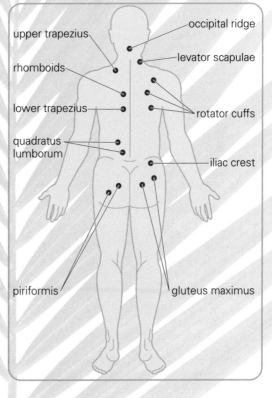

Areas of trigger points

occasionally, as a result of a family predisposition to the condition. Regardless of its development, there are common features that you will see when massaging a person who has kyphosis. First, their pectoral muscles will be very tight and are often in spasm because they have been hunching forward for so long. Similarly, some of the neck muscles will also be in spasm, as they often have a tendency to stick their chin out. While they will complain about pain in their trapezius and

massage in essence

Kyphosis

muscles are linked to underlying bones. For best effects, start the treatment with your partner lying on her back, with a pillow under her spine. This will provide additional softness to increase her comfort, as well as assisting gravity to stretch out the pectoral muscles by pushing the shoulder joints back into the couch. Make sure you do additional effleurage around the sternum and shoulders, and more knuckling to the tops of the shoulders and pectorals. When you turn your partner over to do the back, you can proceed as usual.

Can massage improve scoliosis?
Yes, it can, particularly if the scoliosis is the result of abnormal muscle development. Scoliosis is characterized by an s-shaped or side-to-side curvature of the spine. In milder cases it can be treated effectively with massage or the physical manipulations offered by osteopathy and chiropractic. In more severe cases, the person with scoliosis may require an operation and have pins placed in the spine to help it stabilize. Where the scoliosis has developed because of particular muscle development or overuse – for example, in athletes whose sport involves a range of movements that emphasize one side of the body (javelin, discus and shot-put throwers, as well as

rhomboid muscles, when you work these areas you will most likely find that the muscles are stretched and relatively relaxed, apart from specific nodules of pain at the attachment points where the

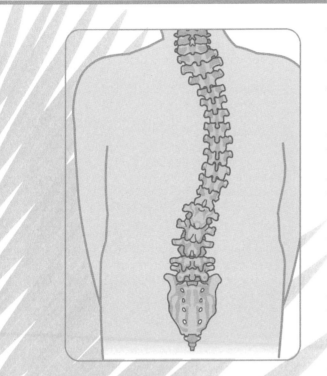

Scoliosis

rowers) – massage can improve the condition. When treating someone who has scoliosis you have to concentrate on the areas where the muscles are over-constricted. Knuckling, kneading and stretching to the over-constricted muscles is particularly useful.

What can I do to help my son? He has cystic fibrosis and the physiotherapist has told me that I will need to massage him regularly.

The physiotherapist will give you precise instructions about how you can use massage to effectively clear the catarrh which develops in your son's chest. Most of the treatment will probably involve cupping (see page 57). You can use this movement to help clear catarrh by having your son lie face down, with his hips across a pillow (or across your knees if he is still small). Having his hips raised will put his back at an angle which will make it easier for him to bring up any catarrh which is in his lungs. You will have to do a lot of cupping (usually anywhere upwards of ten minutes per day) to get the best effects. Your son will be able to tell you when he feels that the treatment has eased his chest. You may want to vary how and when you do the treatments (perhaps two five-minute treatments a day, for example) to suit your son's needs. This treatment is not only useful for those who suffer from cystic fibrosis; it can also help bring up catarrh in those with coughs characterized by a lot of mucus. However, it is often very uncomfortable for people who suffer from asthma or other chest conditions (especially when they are stress-related) and is not advised in these cases.

abdomen

Abdominal massage is another area that tends to be neglected, which is a great shame, given that it is very effective at supporting digestive complaints, such as IBS, relieving menstrual pain and preventing (as well as improving the appearance of) stretch marks. Abdominal massage is also deeply relaxing, as most people tend to store a great deal of tension in this area – think of those who say they have butterflies in their stomach when they feel nervous, or who complain of stomach ulcers. On a purely superficial note, abdominal massage can help to regulate bowel movements and, if practised regularly, can make a significant improvement to muscle tone in the area.

Deep abdominal massage

Contraindication note: this treatment is to be avoided during pregnancy and the first three days of menstruation.

1 Expose belly to xiphoid process and down to hips. Apply oil.

2 Circular effleurage.

3 Lateralizing effleurage.

4 Kneading to waist area (anterior serratus, transverse abdominis and external obliques), first on opposite side and then on the side closest to where you are standing.

115

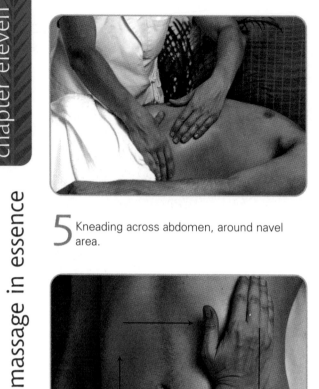

5 Kneading across abdomen, around navel
area.

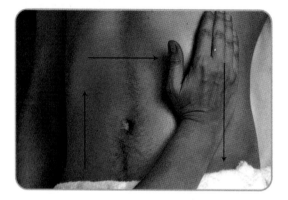

6 Heel-of-hand drainage to colon area – this is
designed to use pressure to clear any toxins
or faecal matter retained in the bowel.
Movements should always be towards the
sigmoid colon. Drain as follows:

• descending colon – splenic flexure to sigmoid
flexure;

• transverse colon – hepatic flexure to splenic
flexure, and then on to sigmoid flexure;

• ascending colon – ileocaecal valve to hepatic
flexure, then on to splenic, then sigmoid flexures.

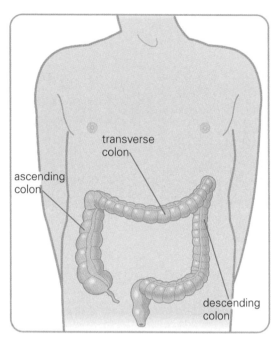

transverse
colon

ascending
colon

descending
colon

7 Repeat, using petrissage to the same areas,
in the same order as drainage with the heel
of the hand.

8 Repeat circular effleurage.

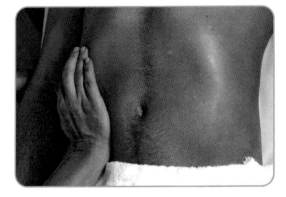

9 Heel-of-hand drainage to liver (ask the client to breathe in, and drain in a 'dog-paddle' style movement as they breathe out).

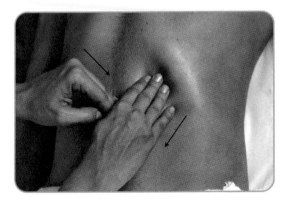

Drain first the liver then the spleen

10 Heel-of-hand drainage to the spleen (ask the client to breathe in, and drain in a 'dog paddle' style movement as they breathe out).

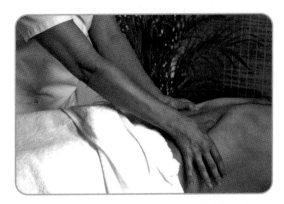

11 Thumb drainage to the diaphragm – put your thumbs at the xiphoid process, ask the client to breathe in, and as they breathe out run your thumbs along the bottom edge of the ribcage.

12 Lateralizing effleurage.

13 Circular effleurage, which gets lighter to finish.

117

FAQs: About abdominal massage

Can massage help to minimize my stretch marks?

Yes, it can, even if it has been some time since you got the stretch marks. For best effects, use calendula as a carrier oil and cover the whole area, massaging slowly until the oil has been absorbed. You can also get very good results if you add certain essential oils to the carrier oil you are using. See *Aromatherapy in Essence* (in the same series as this book, also published by Hodder Arnold) for details. If you are currently pregnant, start massaging plain calendula oil into your skin now to lower your chances of getting stretch marks.

Abdominal massage has helped to relieve some of the pain I get when I menstruate. Can I do anything else to make the massage more effective?

Warmth also helps with the pain relief. Try having a warm bath before your massage and using a hot-water bottle on your abdomen or lower back after the treatment.

I have an inguinal hernia which happened when I tore something playing football. Is it safe for me to massage my abdomen?

You really need to talk to your doctor about this, especially as I assume that you are awaiting an operation.

I am a bit embarrassed in massage class because sometimes when someone massages my abdomen, I get an erection.

I am really not interested in the other people in class sexually. What can I do?

This is a completely normal reaction, as it indicates that you find the massage relaxing. The nervous system has two key ways of causing change in the body – sympathetic nerve action, which speeds things up (the accelerator), and parasympathetic nerve action (the brakes). When parasympathetic nerve action is in force and the body is relaxing, one of the things that happens is that sexual function is increased (so people are more interested in sex when they are relaxed, and, even if they are not interested in sex right at that minute, their bodies can sometimes make it plain that sex is a possibility).

There are a couple of things you can do in situations like this. If you feel able to discuss it with your classmates, you might want to suggest that they apply more pressure during the abdominal massage (sometimes if the pressure is too light it can seem like more of a caress than a therapeutic treatment). Another option is to make some excuse about how you do not want an abdominal massage at that point (a recent meal? you want more work done on your back?). Whichever approach you take, remember that this particular section of the massage seems to have a very relaxing effect on you. Even if you do not have an abdominal massage in class, massage yourself in this area at home, as it will really make a difference to your personal health and stress levels.

the face

Over the years I have found facial massage to be one of the most popular treatments with clients. We tend not to spend a great deal of time working the face outside of the massage class, perhaps because a home beauty routine does not always include much more than the application of a moisturizer. Receiving a facial treatment can feel incredibly luxurious, not least because you are lying down, having your face properly cleaned and having all the delicate muscles treated with care and consideration. Often it is not until someone spends the time (often as much as an hour)

doing a facial treatment that you start to notice just how much tension you hold in your face – muscles to grit your teeth with (or grind them), muscles to keep smiling over, muscles involved in frowning (both if you are unhappy and if your eyesight is not what it used to be), and so much more. The routine suggested here can take between ten minutes and an hour to complete, depending on what you want to achieve. If the person you are treating really needs to relax, add in extra effleurage and spend a lot of time doing the petrissage and the movements over the scalp. Enjoy!

Facial routine

1 Apply oil to the face.

2 Effleurage the face. Keep this rhythmic, gentle and flowing, from chin to ears, chin to temples, then from the chin, around the mouth, up the sides of the nose and across the forehead. Return to the chin and repeat the movement.

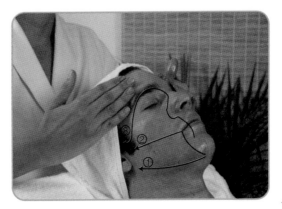

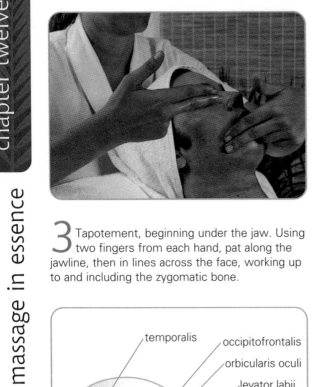

3 Tapotement, beginning under the jaw. Using two fingers from each hand, pat along the jawline, then in lines across the face, working up to and including the zygomatic bone.

temporalis

occipitofrontalis

orbicularis oculi

levator labii superior alaeque nasi

levator labii superioris

zygomaticus

buccinator

orbicularis oris

depressor labii inferioris

depressor anguli oris

masseter

sternoceidomastoid

4 Repeat effleurage.

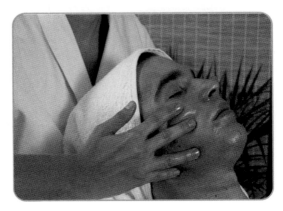

5 Lymph drainage (raking movement) to lower part of the face, drawing lymph towards the nodes in front of the ears.

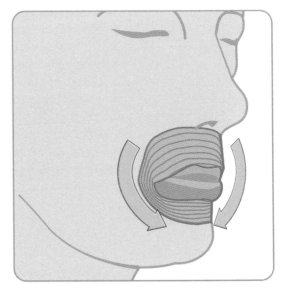

6 Using fingertips, circular stroking around the mouth (orbicularis oris).

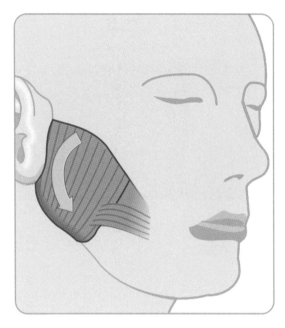

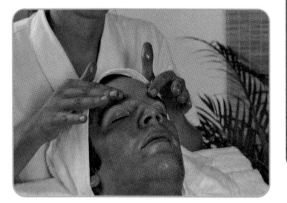

11 Gentle pressure with thumbs along the eyebrow – take the movement to the temples and rotate gently. Repeat.

7 Work on masseter muscle – circular pressures with fingertips over muscle.

8 Repeat effleurage to entire face.

9 Massage ears.

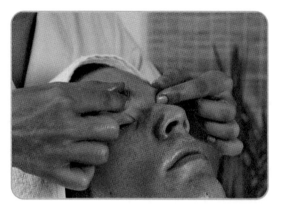

12 Pinch out along eyebrow from inner brow, stroke to temple.

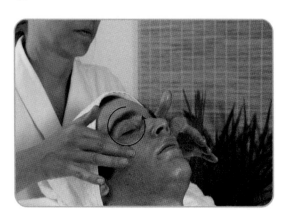

10 Circular strokes around eyes, taking movements out towards the temples, rotating with light pressure at the temples.

121

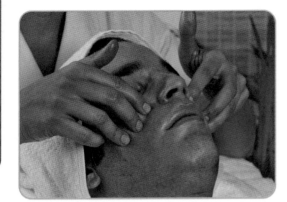

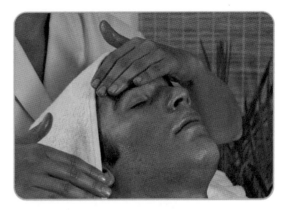

13 Pressure and tapping over sinuses around eyebrows and under the zygomatic arch.

14 Alternate stroking with palm over forehead.

15 Effleurage to finish.

casestudy: Dropping years from your face

Janet, who is in her mid-fifties, works as an advisory teacher and enjoys gardening and golf. Both her hobbies keep her outside a lot, which, in conjunction with a stressful job, has meant that her skin began to suffer. She developed quite dry, papery skin that she felt was making her look older than her years, especially around her throat and neck.

As well as receiving a facial treatment once a month, Janet was advised to start using oil to moisturize her face, replacing her existing cream moisturizers with avocado oil. Although it took her a while to get used to the oil – she only needed a small amount and it was important to allow it time to sink into her skin before applying make up – Janet noticed dramatic changes to the quality and appearance of her skin within six weeks. These changes were so noticeable that even her husband started to use her facial oils in the hope that he too would look younger. She continues to use oil on her face and now takes the time to massage her face once or twice a week, as well as just applying oil on a twice-daily basis.

FAQs: About facial massage

I have oily skin which is prone to acne and I do not feel comfortable about putting more oil on my face. What do you suggest I do?

I know it may seem crazy to add oil to oily skin, but the oil acts as a mild antiseptic and helps to balance out the sebum production in the skin. Specific carrier oils – like jojoba, macadamia nut oil or camellia – are chemically very similar to sebum. When you use these oils as your carrier oil, any dirt or materials which are clogging your pores will dissolve in the oil, making it easier to get dirt out of your pores.

Try to bear with the idea of putting oil on your face and do this daily for a month – you will see a big difference after that time. If you think you would benefit from a cleansing mask first, try using puréed green grapes; leave them on your skin for about five minutes, then wash off with warm water and apply the oil. You can do this mask as often as once a week.

I grind my teeth in my sleep. Can massage help stop me doing this?

To a certain extent it can, although I suspect you would find it more useful to speak to your dentist and get a specialized mouth guard, which will force you to relax the muscles around your jaw when you sleep. If you are using massage alone, then the most effective way of trying to get you to relax your jaw, face, neck and shoulders is to have a very relaxing treatment in the evening before you sleep. Extensive effleurage, kneading and petrissage over the upper back and neck will help to relax stiff muscles that are increasing stress and tension levels. Do not neglect the facial massage, but this time do additional petrissage movements along the sides of the face and jawline. Do the movements first with the mouth shut, then with the jaw open, taking in the buccinator, masseter and temporalis muscles.

developing your own routine

Once you are feeling confident with the various massage movements and you have noticed that you are getting better at recognizing when muscles are tense, if there is inflammation, changes in temperature or similar features, the next step is to go off the path established by the routine you have learned and start to treat the person you are working on holistically – dealing with the situation or symptoms that they arrive with. Sometimes that prospect can be a bit frightening, especially if you are limited in terms of the amount of time you have to treat them or you feel you do not know where to start. In this chapter, we will be looking at some of the things you can do to make developing your own routine easier and more creative.

One of the most valuable tools you can pick up to aid this is the technique of postural analysis. Postural analysis is frequently used by sports massage therapists to identify specific muscle problems their clients have in order to work out where to start their treatment, especially if time is limited. This is very important; although people might come to a massage therapist complaining about pain they are currently experiencing in their shoulders, for example, looking at their posture can give you a very good idea if there are other muscles that may be contracted, which are contributing to the pain they are experiencing.

Postural analysis

1 Start by viewing the person's posture both from the back and the side (with their shoes off), looking particularly for any evidence of spinal curvatures.

   Someone with kyphosis, or dowager's hump, will have a deep curve of their thoracic spine and correspondingly tight muscles in their upper chest area, usually with accompanying tight muscles in the neck area. Plan to start work on their chest muscles before you work other areas.

massage in essence

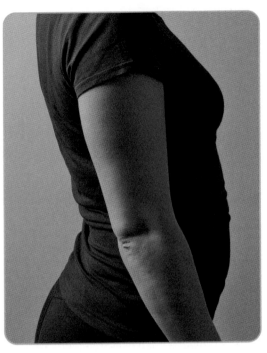

Lordosis

Someone with lordosis, or an exaggerated curve of their lumbar spine, will usually have very tight muscles in the lumbar and gluteal areas and may have correspondingly slack muscles in the abdomen.

Someone with scoliosis will have patterns of contracted and relaxed muscles zigzagging across their body, often starting right down at the knee and going all the way up to the neck. You will need to identify these patterns and work initially away from the area of pain. Start with the legs.

2 Move to the front and look at the angle of their head. Do they tilt their head? Is their chin jutting forward or pulled in and back?

A tilt to the head means that the muscles to one side of the neck are contracted. These are usually the sternocleidomastoid muscles, so they should also have difficulty with step 8,

when you ask them to turn their head to one side. The muscles that are going to be contracted will be the ones on the side where the ear is closest to the shoulder. You will need to do extra work on the neck when they are lying face up. Concentrate on petrissage of the contracted muscle and gentle stretching once the muscles are properly warmed up.

When the chin is habitually jutting forward, it tends to mean that the muscles at the back of the neck and the upper shoulders are over-contracted (splenius capitis, trapezius, levator scapulae). This is quite a common occurrence, especially if someone's eyesight has deteriorated as a result of excessive work on the computer or if they drive a lot.

3 Look at their shoulders. Is one higher than the other?

This is very common. In a woman, it is often an indication that she carries heavy weights on the side where the shoulder is higher (her handbag, a child). In both sexes, it is also occasionally an indication of frequent computer work if they are using a mouse (usually the right shoulder will be higher) or of some form of exercise which involves cross-body stretching or movements. Martial arts, boxing and rowing can all contribute to this. You will need to work on the pectoral muscles (the shoulder will usually be rotated slightly forward) and the trapezius. The rhomboids are likely to be painful and possibly slightly inflamed.

4 If their arms are relaxed by their sides, look at the gap between their arm and their body. Does it seem wider on one side than on the other?

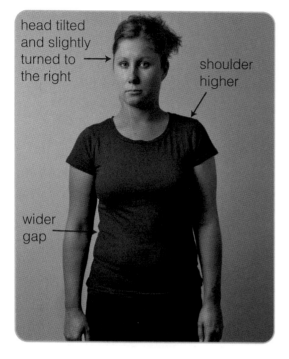

head tilted and slightly turned to the right →

shoulder higher

wider gap

who continually wear high-heeled shoes. This person will need extensive kneading and stretching to the gastrocnemius and soleus.

Flat feet or high arches will give you an indication of muscles that are relatively contracted or relaxed to either the medial (inside) or lateral (outside) portion of the leg (peroneus longus or brevis).

6 If they bend over to touch their toes, how far can they comfortably reach? Do they notice any tight muscles when they do this?

If they are unable to touch their toes and are otherwise fit, this is often an indication of very tight calf muscles (gastrocnemius and soleus) or hamstrings, both of which will benefit from a lot of kneading and possibly knuckling, hacking and cupping. Sometimes there will also be problems with the gluteal muscles.

7 If they bend to one side, then the other, does it seem that one side is more flexible than the other?

This often indicates problems with the gluteals, lumbar muscles, iliopsoas, tensor fasciae latae and also the erector spinae group, especially if they seem to lean slightly forward when they are bending to the side. Kneading and knuckling will be particularly useful, as will slow stretches to the muscles along the lateral sides of the legs and the waist.

8 If they turn their head to one side, then the other, can they turn it further in one direction?

This usually indicates problems with the sternocleidomastoid and also the rest of the cervical muscles, especially if they seem to bring their chin forward in order to turn their head to the side.

This indicates two things: first, the pelvis may be tilted to one side, in which case the lumbar and gluteal muscles will be contracted, especially to one side (and this may have associated pain); second, it indicates that the lumbar and abdominal muscles may well be contracted to one side. Kneading and petrissage movements will be particularly useful, especially over the abdomen.

5 Look at their feet – especially at the arches and at the ankles. Are they flat-footed? Do they have high arches? Can they comfortably rest their heels on the ground?

Looking at their feet will give you a very clear idea of any problems with the calf muscles. The person who cannot rest their heels comfortably on the ground will be someone who has a relatively short Achilles tendon and a very tight gastrocnemius. This is most commonly seen in women

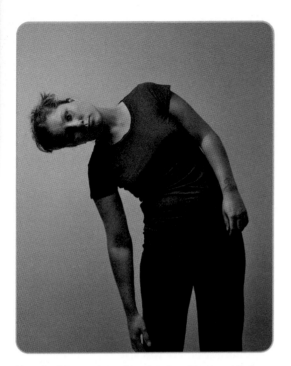

How flexible are they when they bend to one side then the other?

Once you have carried out the postural analysis, your next step would be to ask questions relating to what you see. Is the client aware of pain or tight muscles in the areas that you have identified? Is it a result of an accident or recent injury? Has anything happened that they can link the problems to? (Do not forget that this could be stress-related.) When you are ready to start the massage, you will be concentrating on the areas where you have noticed tension.

where to go from here

Completing your first course in massage is an important landmark to note, especially as it often means that you find yourself at a crossroads, trying to decide which way to move forward. Your options could look something like this:

- stop here and enjoy practising what you have learned;
- carry on and get a professional qualification in massage;
- get a professional qualification in another therapy.

Going no further

If you have enjoyed your course, have learned something and had fun in the process, then it has been a success. People decide to learn massage for a wide variety of reasons; just because you have enjoyed yourself, it does not mean that you *have* to go on to complete your professional training. Remember that there are always a wide variety of short courses you can do that will enhance your skills when you are ready to learn more. Many colleges run introductory courses in all kinds of complementary therapies. If the massage course was enjoyable, but being a massage therapist does not feel quite right to you, try something else (as long as it still feels like fun).

Finding a professional massage course

Massage is easily the most popular therapy for people to learn as they first develop an interest in either complementary therapies or beauty therapy. As a result, professional massage courses are widely available, with the majority of these courses being offered in further education colleges, some higher education colleges (and as part of foundation or undergraduate degree programmes in some universities), community education colleges and in a large number of private colleges. It can be very difficult to choose between the learning establishments, as well as the different courses, so take your time making your decision about how you want to learn and where. You may want to consider the following:

- ☙ When you are available to attend class – most of the courses available through FE colleges are part-time courses, scheduled to take place every week. You would have to set aside at least one evening (or part of a day) per week, usually for about one academic year. Private colleges tend to offer more flexibility in their timing – courses will be available on weekends or as a module, where you would take an intensive course of training prior to sitting your exams.

- ☙ Location and ease of access – you may want to visit the college you will be attending to see how easy it is to get to, as well as to view the training rooms you will be having your classes in. This will often give you a good idea about the facilities the tutor will be using, as well as the variety of resources they will have access to in order to enhance your learning experience.

- ☙ Price – almost without exception, the courses run through FE colleges and community education tend to be cheaper than those run through higher education and private colleges, because the government funds part of the course in order to make it more accessible for new students. However, there are distinct benefits to learning through a private college. Above and beyond the flexibility in timing, you tend to get a very good

standard of teaching (partly because they pay their tutors more), more personal attention in class and often a more informal learning environment. The private colleges may also have a reputation for excellence or additional learning features which would justify the higher fees.

- ☙ Learning support – if you have special educational needs or feel you would benefit from additional support while you are learning, you must raise this with the college you are interested in. All the colleges will have policies about how they address special learning needs, and you will want to check that you are happy with the support you have been promised.

- ☙ How you will be assessed – although all professional massage qualifications in Britain are set at the equivalent of NVQ level 3, there are differences in the methods of assessment used. For example, with certain examining boards, all practical assessment is carried out by your tutor and checked by another tutor in the college. Other examining boards have an external practical examiner who visits the college at the end of your course and watches you (and your classmates) carry out a treatment under timed conditions, as well as asking you specific questions related to your work. Theory assessment, meanwhile, can involve coursework, oral examinations, college-set examinations, externally set and marked examinations, or a combination of the above. These exams can be multiple-choice, short answer or essay questions, depending on the examining board, so even if you are fearful of examinations, remember that your tutor and the college are there to support you and prepare you for your final assessments. If your fear of examinations is particularly debilitating, there are courses that have no external examinations at all. However, there are situations where exams are infinitely preferable to excessive amounts of coursework.

❧ Any added extras – these are most frequently seen in the private colleges, where your course may have a widely recognized qualification embedded within it, but you would be expected to learn additional techniques or theory above and beyond the requirements of the qualification offered. For example, you may choose a massage course which also includes specialist massage techniques or applications, introductory material from another discipline and/or specialist information on subjects such as nutrition, counselling or spiritual healing.

❧ Accreditation of prior learning – each college and examination board will have set different criteria about what they recognize as prior learning that would exempt you from particular sections of the course. For example, whatever course you choose to take, you will be expected to pass examinations in anatomy and physiology. You may want to discuss these with your tutor or with the college if you already hold qualifications in this subject at A level (if taken very recently) or above.

❧ Which professional associations recognize the course – taking a course in massage with the intent to practise as a massage therapist would be a waste of time if, after completing your course, you could not get insurance to practise because the course is not recognized by one of the governing bodies. If you are already aware of and interested in a professional association that you intend to join, visit their website or ask for details about the schools they recommend before making your final decision.

Getting a professional qualification in another therapy

Massage is not always for everyone. You may decide you would prefer one of the following:

❧ A therapy where your client remains clothed – try reflexology, shiatsu or Indian head massage.

❧ One that concentrates on the mind and emotions – consider counselling, life coaching, art or music therapy, or perhaps flower remedies.

❧ One that involves working with the flow of life force or universal energy – perhaps reiki, acupuncture, acupressure, shiatsu, Tui na or Jin Shin Jyutsu.

❧ One that enhances your existing knowledge of massage and allows you to develop more specialized skills – try aromatherapy, acupressure, manual lymphatic drainage, stone therapy, remedial or sports massage.

❧ One that is more academic and has a highly regarded career path within the National Health Service – while massage is widely accepted within a variety of ways of learning, a more academic course might include the training experienced by physiotherapists, osteopaths,

FAQs: About taking massage further

What areas can you work in for massage?
When you are fully qualified, there are opportunities to work as a massage therapist in a wide range of locations and situations. You can work full time or part time; in the day or the evening; from home, as a mobile therapist, in sports centres, beauty salons, health centres, spas, for sports teams, on cruise ships, for airlines, on location for various holiday companies, visiting large businesses, at exhibitions, in a supporting role at large sporting events, in hospice care, for the elderly, for the very young and for everyone in between. The only thing that can prevent you working effectively is a lack of knowledge or education, so get your qualifications first and make sure that you are properly insured to practise.

Do I have to be insured to practise massage?
If you intend to massage members of the public and charge for your services, then yes, not only should you be fully qualified, but you must also hold public liability, professional indemnity and professional liability insurance. Insurance is usually sold to therapists via their professional governing body. Therapists working in a salon on a salaried basis are usually covered by the salon's insurance. Self-employed therapists are expected to have their own insurance.

Which areas are the most profitable to go for?
The most successful therapists I know are the ones who have found ways of building massage into their existing lifestyles or interests. If you know a particular group or organization, or you understand the needs of a specific sector of the public very well, then the chances are that this area would be the most successful for you. Build on your own knowledge and experience and add what you have recently learned in order to make it work.

It usually takes a good 6–18 months to develop a business in complementary therapies which is solvent, let alone profitable. This is probably because most therapists finish their training and start to reinvent the wheel by setting up a practice which does not target a particular group or focus on the experiences and groups the therapist already knows about. Take the time to think carefully about what success

chiropractors or acupuncturists, depending on your personal preferences. In these careers, training starts at degree level and will involve at least three years of learning. Osteopaths, for example, train for five years.

These suggestions are just the beginning of a very long list of treatments you may want to consider. Remember, however, that no learning is ever wasted. Massage, especially a professional qualification in the subject, is often seen as the first step (and possibly a prerequisite) to qualifying in another therapy. For example, it is a requirement alongside or preceding aromatherapy training and is a prerequisite for manual lymphatic drainage or stone therapy qualifications. Some courses do not regard massage as a prerequisite (reflexology, for example), but it can be an advantage.

means to you. For example, success could mean that you set out to treat something specific, such as muscle pain, and your treatment works. Alternatively, if you decide that you will define success as meaning you work one day a week at massage and will be successful if you have three treatments to do in that day, then you will probably feel successful relatively quickly (as long as you do your marketing properly). Proactive marketing and networking which is aimed at a clear group of people will ensure that making a profit will not be quite so far away.

How easy is it to get a job travelling the world doing massage, perhaps working at five-star resorts?

This job is like every other job out there: it sounds glamorous and there will be a lot of positive features to it, but those who have done it would be the first to tell you that there are drawbacks as well. As with any job, there are vacancies which you can apply for (so get your curriculum vitae sorted out), and those vacancies come up fairly regularly. There are a number of magazines, newspapers and internet sites that holiday companies use to advertise for staff. If you do not see advertisements, that does not necessarily mean the jobs are not available. It is often worth sending a covering letter with your CV to the relevant person in the holiday company's personnel department. Start by identifying the company or resort you are interested in working for, visit their website, get a telephone number of someone involved in recruiting staff, and phone them to check who you should send your letter and CV to.

Unless the resort or spa specializes in massage treatments, you will be more interesting to the company as a potential member of staff if you are qualified in more than one discipline. If massage is your first qualification, you may want to consider adding one or more complementary therapies and/or completing beauty therapy qualifications.

How do you build a personal practice? How do you get contacts for new clients?

These questions lead you off to another book altogether and are best addressed once you are well on the way to finishing your professional training. Try *Business Practice for Therapists* by this author (also published by Hodder Arnold).

133

Useful contacts

Finding a massage course

www.hotcourses.com (accessed
27 November 2005)
www.itecworld.co.uk (accessed 27 November
2005)
www.vtct.org.uk (accessed 27 November
2005)

Buying protective clothing

www.dk-profashion.co.uk (accessed
27 November 2005)
www.vitalitywear.co.uk (accessed
27 November 2005)
www.salonsdirect.com (accessed
27 November 2005)

Buying a massage couch

The following offer standard and professional
massage couches at mid-range prices:

Beautelle
www.beautelle.co.uk (accessed
27 November 2005)
0121 322 0920

Marshcouch
14 Robinsfield, Hemel Hempstead HP1
1RW
www.marshcouch.com (accessed
27 November 2005)
01442 263199
nigel@marshcouch.com

New Concept
www.new-concept.co.uk (accessed
27 November 2005)
01473 720572

The Massage Table Store
http://massagetablestore.com (accessed
27 November 2005)
01454 261900
020 8983 9800

Glossary

Achilles tendon: the tendon that connects the gastrocnemius (calf muscle) to the calcaneus (heel bone).

Acne rosacea: a variety of acne which usually occurs in a person's late twenties or early thirties, involving broken capillaries on the cheeks, nose and forehead, a tendency to blush easily and a persistent redness to the skin, even if pimples are not visible on the surface.

Acne vulgaris: more commonly regarded as 'teenage' acne – even if it is not exclusive to the young – involving inflamed pus-filled lesions which can occur anywhere on the body, but most frequently appear on the face, neck, back and chest.

Acromion process: the bony prominence at the joint of the clavicle and the scapula.

Acupressure: pressure-point massage.

Adductors: muscles at the top of the inner thigh – the adductors magnus, brevis and longus help to press the thighs together and are important in walking. These muscles are strained if you have a 'pulled groin'.

Adrenaline: a hormone produced by the adrenal glands, sometimes called epinephrine, which initiates the body's response to stress. Its effects include raised heart rate, raised blood pressure, increased blood supply to the heart, brain, lungs and skeletal muscles, and dilation of the bronchial tubes in the lungs.

Anorexia: an eating disorder characterized by an obsessive desire to lose weight by refusing to eat.

Antibacterial: a substance which kills bacteria.

Anti-fungal: a substance which kills fungal or yeast infections.

Anti-inflammatory: a substance which reduces inflammation.

Antiseptic: kills bacteria and microbes.

Aromatherapy: a treatment which involves the application of essential oils, usually including massage.

Arthritis: pain, stiffness and swelling of the joints.

Athlete's foot: a fungal infection, sometimes known as tinea pedis, which appears almost exclusively on the feet, usually between the toes.

Ayurvedic: deriving from the study of Ayurveda, a system of healing originating in India.

Buccinator: a facial muscle that is used in smiling when you move the corners of your mouth outwards.

Bulimia: an eating disorder which involves binge eating followed by some activity which is designed to purge the system (this may include vomiting, using laxatives and/or diuretics, and excessive exercise).

Carpals: the eight bones of the wrist – scaphoid, lunate, triquetral, pisiform, trapezium, trapezoid, capitate and hamate.

Cervical: the neck region of the spine. There are seven cervical vertebrae.

Colic: digestive discomfort common in very young infants (it usually disappears by the time

135

they are around three months old) involving painful trapped wind. The infant will cry and draw his/her legs up to the belly when experiencing colic.

Contraindication: a presenting symptom or disorder that prevents treatment or makes it inadvisable to practise as you would normally (you may choose to continue to treat, but might avoid working on certain areas or doing certain massage movements).

Coracobrachialis: a small muscle which is involved in flexing the humerus and moving it closer to the body.

Cortisol: a hormone produced by the adrenal glands which is involved in the body's response to stress; it encourages the body to use fat and protein to create sugar, saving any sugar for use by the brain during a stressful situation. Cortisol enhances the effects of adrenaline, especially in raising blood pressure.

Cross-infection: to pass an infection from one part of the body to another or from one body to another.

Cubital crease: the medial (or inner side) of the elbow.

Cystic fibrosis: a genetic disease which is eventually fatal. Symptoms include a thick mucus which fills the respiratory passages and needs to be 'clapped' or cupped out.

Cytophylactic: encourages healthy cell growth.

Deep-vein thrombosis: a blood clot found in the deep, large veins, usually of the legs. If the clot is large enough, it can block circulation to cells beyond the clot, causing cell death.

Deltoids: the muscles which lie on the shoulder and take the arm away from the body when they contract. They are active when you swing your arms.

Dermatitis: inflammation of the dermal region of the skin.

Diabetes: a disorder related to the supply of insulin by the pancreas. People with diabetes do not make enough insulin to meet their body's needs. Type I diabetes involves the person injecting themselves with insulin at least four times a day. Type II diabetes involves controlling your blood sugar levels through diet (and occasionally the tablet form of insulin).

Dopamine: a neurotransmitter which makes you 'feel good'. It is supposedly deficient in someone who has Parkinson's disease and it may be involved in the development of schizophrenia in some patients.

Dysmenorrhoea: painful menstrual periods.

Eczema: skin disorder which involves an allergic-type response to a substance which has either been exposed to the skin or has been eaten. It is often made worse by stress. It usually results in weeping (or bleeding) sores which are intensely itchy.

Effleurage: flowing massage movement which is used to start and finish most massage treatments.

Endometriosis: painful condition in which the endometrial tissue lining the uterus migrates to other parts of the abdominal cavity.

Epilepsy: Seizures which occur as a result of abnormal electrical discharge in the brain. These can develop as a result of a family history of the disorder as well as a blow to the head, infection, high fever or a tumour.

Erector spinae: a group of muscles extending all the way along the spine, which help to keep the back erect and to control the movement when you bend forward to touch your toes.

External obliques: muscles in lower waist area, which aid the back muscles in rotating the trunk and doing side-bends.

Fascia lata: muscle in the lateral portion of the thigh which helps to flex and abduct the thigh (taking it out from the body) and is also involved in rotating the thigh inwards.

Femur: the thigh bone.

Gastrocnemius: main calf muscle (gives the top of the calf its characteristic bulging shape), which is involved in flexing the foot and pointing the toes.

Gluteus maximus: the largest of the gluteal muscles, which is working when you push the thigh backwards as you are climbing stairs or when you are running.

Gluteus medius: the middle gluteal muscle, which is most active in walking.

Gluteus minimus: the smallest and deepest of the gluteal muscles, which works with the gluteus medius.

Gracilis: long muscle on the inside of the thigh, which helps to bring the thigh inwards and is involved in walking.

Hamstrings: a group of three muscles at the back of the thigh – the semimembranosus, semitendinosus and biceps femoris.

Hernia: a protrusion of part of an organ (usually the intestine) through a wall of the cavity in which it is normally enclosed.

Holistic: an approach to treatment which takes into consideration the body, mind, emotions and spirit of the individual, as well as their environment.

Humerus: the bone of the upper arm.

Huna: form of massage developed in Hawaii.

Hypertension: high blood pressure, usually above 175/100.

Hypoallergenic: non-allergic.

Iliotibial band: a thickened portion of the fascia lata which extends from the top of the hip to the knee.

Impetigo: a bacterial skin infection forming pustules and yellow crusty sores. It is highly contagious.

Infraspinatus: muscle which lies over the shoulder and is partially covered by the deltoids and the trapezius. It helps to hold the humerus (the bone of the upper arm) in its joint and is involved in rotating the arm.

Inguinal: of the groin region.

Irritable bowel syndrome: disorder of the bowels which usually results in alternating constipation and diarrhoea.

Kneading: massage movement which involves passing flesh from one hand to the other in a rhythmic manner.

Knuckling: massage movement which involves the knuckles of the therapist's hands pressing and rotating over large areas of muscle.

Kyphosis: exaggerated curvature of the thoracic spine, sometimes referred to as 'dowager's hump'.

Latissimus dorsi: triangular muscle of the lower back which is involved in extending the arm, rotating it at the shoulder. Involved in swimming, rowing or any movement which involves bringing the arm down forcefully.

Ligaments: tough fibrous tissues which joins ankles together and hands together.

Lordosis: exaggerated curvature of the lumbar region of the spine, most often found in pregnant women, those who have gained weight suddenly and in certain athletic disciplines.

Lumbar: of the lower back and waist region.

Lymph: the liquid portion of blood (plasma) which escapes from the cardiovascular system to bathe the cells of nearby tissues.

Lymph nodes: lymphatic tissue occurring in various parts of the body where lymph is filtered and lymphocytes are formed.

Masseter: muscle of the face which helps to close the jaw.

Menorrhagia: heavy periods.

Metastasize: to move (usually of cancer cells), this means that the cancer has moved and will grow elsewhere.

Metatarsals: five bones found in each foot.

Myalgic encephalomyelitis: muscle and nerve pain and exhaustion, usually following a viral reaction.

Neuralgia: nerve pain.

Neurotransmitters: chemical substances used by the nervous system to assist in the passage of messages.

Noradrenaline: hormone produced by the adrenal glands which is involved in the body's response to stress.

Oedema: water retention, which can appear anywhere, but is most likely to develop in the lower limbs, around the abdomen or occasionally in the hands and arms.

Oestrogen: a hormone produced by the ovaries, linked to the development of fertile eggs in women and closely related to the development of female physical characteristics.

Oleocranon process: bony prominence at the elbow.

Osteoarthritis: arthritis which develops as a result of wear and tear on the joints.

Osteoporosis: a condition of the bones which involves them starting to crumble as a result of a loss of calcium. The condition is most common in the elderly, although it can develop in younger people, especially in those women who may cease to menstruate for a while (perhaps as a result of sudden weight loss, over-exercise or similar). It is usually linked to poor eating habits, insufficient exercise, smoking and/or alcohol intake.

Palmar: of the palm of the hand.

Parasympathetic: nerve action which slows down the body's processes, lowering blood pressure and heart rate, increasing digestive action and encouraging sleep.

Peak airflow: sometimes called the vital capacity, this is the maximum amount of air which can be breathed out after taking a deep breath in.

Pectorals: muscles across the top of the chest.

Perineum: area of muscle between the vagina and the anus.

Peristalsis: gentle, wave-like contractions which help to move food down the gastrointestinal tract.

Petrissage: a range of grinding movements which usually involves the pressing of muscles into the bones underlying them.

Phlebitis: inflammation of the blood vessels.

Piriformis: a muscle found deep beneath the gluteals which joins the sacrum to the head of the femur and is usually related to problems with sciatica.

Plasma: the liquid portion of blood.

Popliteal: region at the back of the knee, usually associated with the lymph node found there.

Post-viral fatigue: a range of symptoms, including overwhelming exhaustion, which follows a viral infection. This can take many weeks (or months) to recover from.

Progesterone: female hormone produced by the ovaries which is responsible for the development of the lining of the uterus (high levels of progesterone are required to maintain a pregnancy and are believed to be the cause of premenstrual tension symptoms).

Psoriasis: inflammatory skin condition.

Quadriceps: group of four muscles in the front of the thigh – the rectus femoris, vastus lateralis, vastus medialis and vastus intermedius.

Radius: one of the bones of the forearm.

Reflexology: acupressure massage of the feet and hands.

Repetitive strain injury: painful muscle strain, usually to the wrists and hands, caused by overuse of the muscles and joints in the area.

Raynaud's syndrome: a cardiovascular disorder which results in very poor circulation to the hands, feet and skin, often linked to stress.

Rheumatoid arthritis: characterized by pain, stiffness and swelling of the joints, this form of arthritis is an autoimmune condition and most often develops around the age of 35.

Rhomboids: muscles lying between the scapula (shoulder blade) and the spine which pull the scapula towards the spine.

Ringworm: a fungal infection which results in distinctive, itchy, circular patches appearing on the surface of the skin, usually on the scalp or the feet. It is highly contagious.

Sacral: of the sacrum (the triangular bone in the lower back, located between the hip bones of the pelvis).

Scabies: a contagious skin disease caused by a spider-like mite which burrows into the skin, producing raised, itchy, red spots.

Sciatica: pain and inflammation of the sciatic nerve (a major nerve extending from the lower end of the spinal cord down the back of the thigh). This can extend all the way down the leg.

Scoliosis: an s-shaped curvature of the spine.

Sebum: oily substance produced by the skin to help lubricate it effectively.

Serotonin: a neurotransmitter.

Shiatsu: acupressure massage originating in Japan.

Soleus: muscle found in the posterior calf.

Sports massage: style of massage designed to effectively support athletes – either pre- or post-event – to warm up and warm down, and/or in the recovery of sports-related injuries.

Sprain: damage to the ligaments around a joint.

Sternocleidomastoid: muscle of the neck which attaches to the sternum and the clavicle and allows the head to rotate.

Stone therapy: massage using hot and cold stones.

Strain: damage to muscle or tendons, usually as a result of overuse.

Sub-fertility: condition wherein the individual has difficulty conceiving or procreating.

Subscapularis: muscle under the shoulder blade.

Supraspinatus: muscle found at the top of the shoulder blade.

Sympathetic: nerve action which speeds up the body's processes, including raising blood pressure and heart rate.

Tapotement: range of percussion movements used in Swedish, holistic and therapeutic massage.

Temporalis: a fan-shaped muscle running from the side of the skull to the back of the lower jaw.

Tendon: the elastic portion at the end of a muscle which attaches it to a bone.

Teres major: one of the muscles crossing the scapula which is involved in rotating the shoulder.

Teres minor: one of the muscles crossing the scapula which is involved in rotating the shoulder and holds the humerus (bone of the upper arm) in its joint.

Testosterone: hormone produced in the testes, responsible for the development of secondary sexual characteristics in males (including development of skeletal muscle and growth of body hair and beard).

Therapeutic massage: style of massage using the techniques of Swedish massage, with movements towards the heart to improve circulation of blood and lymph.

Thrombosis: a blood clot.

Thyroxine: hormone produced by the thyroid (a large gland in the neck) which governs metabolic rate.

Towel management: range of methods used to handle towels in order to protect the modesty of the person receiving the massage and keep them warm during treatment.

Trapezius: main muscle of the upper back.

Tui na: style of massage originating in China.

Tumour: overgrowth of cells which can be benign or malignant.

Ulna: one of the two bones of the forearm.

Venous flow: blood flow along the veins towards the heart.

Varicose veins: condition of the veins which occurs when blood pools in this area and causes the walls of the veins to distend.

Verrucae: warts found on the base (plantar surface) of the foot.

Warts: small, hard, benign growths on the skin, caused by a virus.

Xiphoid process: small bony prominence at the lower end of the sternum.

index